ALL YOU CAN DO IS DO WHAT YOU MUST: LIVING WITH PARKINSON'S DISEASE

A MEMOIR
by IRA FRIED

Dedication

I dedicate this book to Joy, my wife of thirty-three years and counting.

Parkinson's Disease has changed Joy's life no less than it has changed mine. She has taken on her new role as caregiver with grace and aplomb. She has laughed with me when we needed some humor to break through the despair, held my hand when the pain from my peripheral neuropathy has been too much to bear, and shown me compassion when I needed to know that someone cared about me.

Joy has a deep reservoir of love she gladly shares with her clients, her many friends, Alan and Sam, our cat, Nina, and me. I feel incredibly lucky to be in her orbit.

Note to Reader

In writing an autobiographical memoir, it is impossible not to make oneself the hero of the story. But outside the pages of this book, I realize that I am no hero. The real heros to me are people who put their lives on the line to help others, like the first-responders at 9/11 or people who find places for the homeless to stay.

The characterizations and events described in this book reflect my own interpretation of what has happened during the course of my life. In a few of my vignettes, I have made some minor changes to the sequence of events to make the story more coherent. I have changed many of the names in the book to protect privacy of the innocent and not-so-innocent.

This book is not intended to provide medical advice about Parkinson's or any other disease. Rather, it is an accounting of my intellectual and emotional journey with Parkinson's. I wrote it with the hope that others with medical conditions similar to mine would see that they are not alone.

CONTENTS

CHAPTER 1
NEEDED: POSITIVE PARKIE

Imagine seeing an ad on Monster.com or Craigslist that stated, "Needed: Positive Parkie—an otherwise healthy man in his late forties to become afflicted with early-onset Parkinson's, peripheral neuropathy, and cancer. Interested applicants must demonstrate an ability to maintain a positive attitude as his diseases progress. He must recognize and, with time, accept the changes brought on by his diseases. And he must possess a willingness to accept help in whatever form it comes.

The successful candidate will receive a full range of benefits, including early retirement, plenty of time for introspection, discovering latent talent, and most important, making new friends and strengthening bonds with existing friends and family.

The Positive Parkie must demonstrate an ability for and interest in writing about his experiences. Humor is appreciated but not required. In lieu of a resume we ask candidates to answer the following questions. "What are your core beliefs? How did you come by them? How do you expect these beliefs to help you perform the duties of the position? What skills and/or personality traits do you possess that will enable you to continue to remain positive, at least in public, as your diseases progress? Describe the circumstances that led you to develop these personality traits. Cite a specific example of an unexpected act of kindness that gave you the strength to make it through a difficult time.

The form of your answers is unimportant. Poetry, novel, short story, and memoir are all acceptable. What matters most is the content of your answers. The successful candidate will provide as much or as little information about his life as is needed to make a compelling case that he is the right person for the job.

The candidate shall report directly to his spouse or significant other. Her decisions are final. No arguing. As his disease progresses he will become increasingly dependent on her and she will take on the additional responsibility of caregiver. She will receive an occasional thank you, but no other remuneration for this additional work."

I got the job, or more accurately, the job got me. I had no choice in the matter so I am trying to make the best of it.

. . . .

For the first four years, I excelled at the job. I maintained a positive attitude in public no matter how bad I felt. And, truth be told, I felt good most of the time. Yes, I lost some things I held dear. But I didn't miss them as much as I thought I would. I just calmly watched them recede into the past.

People treated me with respect bordering on reverence. One day some years ago, at the check-out counter of a local diner, I ran into a man I recognized as a neighbor, but otherwise could not place. He said hello and told me his name. With that I remembered him as the parent of one of my younger son's friends from elementary school. I also recalled he was a former professional hockey player.

Before I could return his greeting he told me he saw me almost every day riding my bike, power walking, or running around the neighborhood. He then said that, as a former athlete, he knew how hard it was to push myself the way I do. I tried to object but he continued, saying that seeing me out there day after day was inspirational and I was a hero to him. Then he paid his bill and walked out without uttering another word.

At first, I didn't understand any of what my neighbor had said. I just continued to do what I had always done—work out every day. I didn't see anything heroic in that. The real heroes to me were people who put their lives on the line to help others, like the first-responders at 9/11 or people who find places for the homeless to stay.

But gradually I let his words seep into my consciousness. I started to believe that just going about my day did make me special. I even began to wonder whether Parkinson's, rather than being a disability, gave me an advantage in life.

Meanwhile, Parkinson's and peripheral neuropathy marched relentlessly through my brain, destroying neurons as they advanced. I continued with my life, ignoring the damage my diseases had already done.

Virgil, the name I had given to my cane, had become practically an appendage of my body. My peripheral neuropathy pain episodes came on more frequently, lasted longer, and were more painful than they had ever been. But within a couple of hours of each episode I would almost forget I ever had one. The illnesses had begun to ravage my body while I remained in a state of ignorant (willful?) bliss. My job as a Positive Parkie could not have been going better.

Four years and a little more than a month after I received the Parkinson's diagnosis, I hit my first major bump in the road—my last day of work at Thomson Reuters. I came home that day, my feet moving in a slow shuffle, back stooped and eyes fixed a few feet in front of me. I had planned for this day for five years, but now that it was upon me it felt unreal. My shuffling gait and stooped back signified moderate to severe Parkinson's. My heightened anxiety was likely a side-effect of one of the numerous medications I took each day. I had become a full-time Positive Parkie.

My supervisor—a.k.a. Joy, my wife of over 30 years— calmed me down. She told me that now I was free to do whatever I wanted. "Do whatever will make you happy," she said. "Just don't hang out around the house moping all day."

Joy should have known better. Staying home and feeling sorry for myself is not in my DNA. I joined three not-for-profit boards of directors and quickly took a leadership position in each of them. I provided analytical support to an attorney I had met at Panera's who was leading a class action law suit against one of the Big Pharma drug companies. And I started writing this memoir.

All this within the first years of leaving my job, I crowed. Once again, I thought, I had conquered my diseases. My condition may have worsened, but I found a way to be more productive than ever before. I had fought tougher battles during my childhood, I reasoned. And I had running. Since the age of fourteen, I'd used running as an escape. I'd learned to push myself to run as fast as I could and then even harder, discovering I had more in my reserve than I thought. My intellect, hard work, and refusal to give up had always won out. Why should that not be the case with Parkinson's?

. . . .

Underlying my story of resilience is a cycle of denial, hubris, acceptance, and humility. Time after time I think I have figured it all out only to discover how much I don't know or understand. Denial has been a salve, but it has its limits. I can deny only until circumstances force me to accept the truth.

With acceptance comes humility. I have learned to accept help in ways I had not conceived of before. But then another horrible truth comes lurking around the corner. I can hide this truth too—for a time—with denial. But I know that this truth, like the last, will eventually come into full view.

I have gone through this cycle countless times, starting in my early childhood. Over the years, I have become increasingly adept at recognizing it. With experience, developing a measure of wisdom. Nevertheless, I allow myself to go through this cycle over and over again. As a child I went back to school each day, no matter how bad the taunting the previous day. And as an adult with three degenerative diseases, I refuse to let worries of what tomorrow might bring stop me from living a full and productive life today.

This story is about living with progressive diseases—in my case Parkinson's Disease (PD) and peripheral neuropathy—and how my childhood experiences prepared me to cope with them. (I also have had two cancer scares: a large mass in my right kidney which proved to be benign when the kidney was removed, and an indolent strain of lymphoma, which my oncologist has said will not require treatment for the foreseeable future.)

My memoir is not a day-to-day account of my life with PD and peripheral neuropathy. Instead, it is about the intellectual and emotional journey I have taken as my diseases have advanced. Some of what I wrote may be upsetting or even shocking to some readers. But I believe that only by giving a full, open, and honest account of my inner life can others afflicted with progressive, degenerative diseases benefit from reading this book.

Some readers may question why I have devoted so many pages to my childhood for a memoir about an adult coping with illness. My answer: my childhood tells the story of how I learned to cope with adversity and how resilience became a habit for me. Early in life I started formulating answers to questions I believe everyone saddled with a progressive disease asks him- or herself at one time or another. Questions like: *Why me? How do I cope with a life with so much uncertainty? How can I continue to make my life meaningful?* Not including my childhood in this memoir reduces the answers to these questions to mere clichés.

And so my story begins.

CHAPTER 2
ALBERT AND ANNETTE

We are all, to some extent, a product of our upbringings and that is no less true of Albert and Annette. To understand how they came to be the persons I knew as my father and mother, it is necessary to know a little about their backgrounds.

My Jewish Ancestry

Albert and Annette were both children of Polish Jews who had immigrated to the United States in the early 1900s. My mother's mother and both of my father's parents came to the United States as teenagers. My mother's father, who was at least a decade older than my grandmother, came to the United States as a young adult.

As was generally the case in Europe, the Jews in Poland were segregated from the rest of the population. They spoke a different language, had different religious and cultural traditions, and even followed a different set of laws. They made up a significant portion of the population, especially in the larger cities, and played an integral role in the local economies, but were never a part of Polish society. During good economic times the Jewish people in Poland were allowed to live peaceably. But during bad times, they became scapegoats. They were frequently subjected to pogroms, during which gangs of thugs vandalized the Jewish communities, killing or injuring anyone in their path. Dreams of living in a place where they could be part of the larger society and not live in constant fear of being attacked were important motivators for many Jews who emigrated from Poland to the United States at this time.

While Albert and Annette shared a common Eastern European Jewish heritage, they came from very different socioeconomic strata. As adults, their Jewish heritage remained an essential part of Albert's and Annette's identities. Marrying a non-Jew would have been inconceivable to either of them. In each of the places my family lived as I was growing up, socially, my parents were part of the Jewish community. As far as I can recall, all of their friends were also Jewish. And both of them spoke Yiddish, which they did whenever they didn't want my sisters or me to know what they were talking about.

In many respects the parents I remember from my early childhood perfectly fit the stereotype of the upwardly mobile Jewish-American couple. My mother had her weekly Mahjong game, my father played handball at the Jewish Community Center every Sunday morning, they both loved Chinese food, and they both were very liberal politically.

Annette

Annette Sarah Stern was born in 1931. She grew up in the Bronx near the Grand Concourse, a tree-lined boulevard that in its heyday was described as the Champs Elysees of the Bronx. A 2009 article in the *The New York Times* stated this street was considered "the ultimate prestige address for the vast numbers of the city's upwardly mobile Jews."The surrounding neighborhoods were solidly middle class. This vibrant and safe neighborhood was still considered a very desirable place to live when my mother grew up there in the 1930s and 1940s. This was well before the white flight of the 1950s and 1960s and the fires of the early seventies gave the neighborhood the bombed-out look I remember when I went to college nearby at Fordham.

I don't know much about my mother's childhood. Her parents had enough money to provide a comfortable middle class life. Her father, a pharmacist, owned a small independent drugstore, where her mother frequently helped out. This was before the advent of chain drug stores and pharmacies in supermarkets, so it was still possible to make a decent living this way.

Annette's family celebrated the Jewish "High Holy" holidays of Rosh Hashanah and Yom Kippur, but otherwise religion was not an important part of their lives. Much more important to them was their involvement with The Workmen's Circle, a secular Jewish organization that was and still is active in human/worker's rights issues.

Annette was an only child until the age of thirteen, when her brother Michael was born. Despite the age difference, the two of them were very close and remained so until Annette's death from congestive heart failure in 2008.

From what I have heard, mostly second-hand, she did not have a happy childhood. Both Edythe and Mandy remember her telling stories about how she suffered ver-

9

bal abuse from her parents. Her mother had experienced several miscarriages before Michael was born and took out her anger and resentment on Annette. Annette's father, who I remember as a kind and gentle man, was not the least bit supportive of Annette, sometimes saying things to her that can only be described as cruel. For example, Mandy recalls hearing an argument between Annette and her mother during which Annette recalled telling her father she was getting married. He replied saying something to the effect of, "Good, with you gone, now we can be a real family." It is easy to see how this upbringing would have contributed to the insecurities she exhibited as an adult.

Nevertheless, Annette was an outgoing child and young adult. Energetic and smart, she was popular among both girls and boys. In the late forties when my mother attended high school, full-figured women like Betty Grable and Jane Russell embodied the ideal of feminine beauty. My mother, with her round face, cherubic nose, and curvy figure, was considered very attractive. A long line of boys at her school wanted to date her.

Annette was a good but not exceptional student. In 1950, the year she graduated from high school, most women from middle class backgrounds did not go to college. To the best of my knowledge, it was not an option for Annette, nor did she aspire to go. Instead, she went to work in an office directly after high school, her first job a low-level clerical position. She gradually took on more responsibility, but never moved up beyond the secretarial pool.

. . . .

Had Annette been born twenty years later, she may well have gone to college. My mother had a thirst for knowledge. An avid reader, mainly of general interest women's magazines and novels, she also kept up on current affairs by reading the local newspaper and watching the evening news every day. She knew a little about a wide range of topics and was proud of what she knew. Her breadth of knowledge was so wide she always had some wisdom to impart, no matter what the topic, frequently telling people about an interesting fact she had recently discovered. She also had strong opinions about the politics of the day, which she was not shy about expressing.

When Annette and my father weren't arguing, they often talked about his work. To my ears it seemed to be mostly about who said what to whom. But it is clear to me now that my mother had taken an interest in and had an understanding of the politics in my father's office. And he must have found her to be helpful as a sounding board because, at least when I was young, he talked to her about his job almost every night.

My mother was also a very good friend. When I was about seven years old, a friend of hers told her that her husband was beating her. My mother became her main confidante and supporter. During one particularly bad time she invited her friend and three children to stay with us. They ended up staying for a week. My mother encouraged her friend to get out of the marriage, and when her friend finally sued for divorce and the case went to court, my mother testified on her behalf. To put this story in perspective, one needs to bear in mind that it happened in the mid-sixties, well before domestic violence became an issue people spoke about in public.

Unfortunately, the person I have lodged in early-child-hood memory as my mother bears only a faint resemblance to the attractive, engaging person I just described. By the time of my first recollection, she had transformed from chubby to obese, and always seemed to be yelling at someone—if not my father, then one of my sisters or me. Outside of our home, she was a gregarious, upbeat person with a wide circle of friends, but inside our home she was mostly just loud and angry. She seemed ready to explode at any moment. And when she did explode, she often became nasty, lashing out at me or one of my sisters with verbal abuse for the slightest offense. Not putting a dirty plate in the dishwasher or spilling something was all it took. During her outbursts she often called me or one of my sisters an "idiot's delight." I would not know what that meant until my teenage years, but her scarlet face and screeching voice made it clear to me, even as a little boy, that it wasn't good. It must be said, however, that no matter how furious my mother got she never once threw or broke anything or hit me or my sisters.

My mother's weight was an unspoken (for us kids) but constant theme that ran like a current through our household. Back then, obesity was not nearly as common as it is today, so my mother really stood out. Once, when I was about six or seven, I got in trouble because she thought I had told someone she was fat. Of course, I did think she was fat, but never would have actually said it. To my mother's credit, she dieted constantly from the time of her break-up with my father until her death. I must have witnessed her lose and then gain back a hundred pounds or more half a dozen times. I sometimes wonder, with regret, whether we would have had something approaching a normal mother-son relationship if only I had realized how much courage it took for her to go on these diets—a heroic act of willpower each time she won a battle, only to fail a few months later. And with everyone in her social group watching. I admire her for the perseverance it must have taken.

This behavior in no way excuses her for the abuse she meted out, but it does call attention to a positive side of her that I did not until recently realize existed. Thinking about my mother's struggles with her weight now, I have to give her credit. She kept trying over and over again to lose weight; she never gave up. I would like to think I inherited some of that determination from her.

Despite all the discord in her relationship with my father, my mother wrapped a good part of her self-identity around being the wife of the rising corporate executive. She was genuinely proud of my father's achievements and enjoyed the lifestyle and status they brought her. She used to refer to General Electric as "Generous Electric." She performed the duties expected of a corporate wife very well. In the early years, in addition to being a sounding board for my father, she got up early every weekday morning to help him get ready for work, often choosing his tie for him, and to make a hot breakfast for him, my sisters, and me. Every evening she had dinner waiting for him when he got home.

Entertaining colleagues and their spouses was an important part of the corporate culture at General Electric, and my mother did this very well too. She could always be counted on to prepare a delicious and creative meal and could carry on an intelligent conversation with her guests, even though many of them were more educated. My mother prided herself on being able to handle events of any size, from dinner with just one other couple to parties with dozens of guests. Even her leadership position at B'nai B'rith was part and parcel of what was expected of a corporate wife.

In 1966, when I was eight years old, my father got a major promotion, which required us to move from Fairfield, Connecticut, to Lexington, Massachusetts. This move must have been difficult for my mother because it meant leaving a large network of friends, including several who were very close. But my mother started right up where she left off. She quickly made new friends and got heavily involved with ORT, a Jewish organization that promotes education and understanding between people of different backgrounds.

Once again, I have to give my mother some credit. She demonstrated the same type of resiliency in dealing with this move that I think has helped me to deal with Parkinson's and peripheral neuropathy. What she was going through then was not all that different from what I am going through today. Whereas I am living with a progressive disease that is causing me to decline physically, she was living in a progressively worsening marriage that was causing her self-confidence to erode. I have no evidence, but little doubt, that my father regularly saw other women by that time and my mother had at least an inkling of my father's infidelity. The hurt and shame must have chipped away at her already frail ego.

Two years after we moved to Lexington, my father got promoted again, requiring a move to Pittsfield, Massachusetts. At the time, Pittsfield was essentially a General Electric company town. My father was one of the top GE executives, and so was widely known. To my mother, it was like living in a fish bowl. She hated it. She did not join any service organizations and no longer got up every morning to help my father get ready for work and make breakfast for the family. The acrimony between her and my father continued to intensify. She was starting to become bitter about what her life had become and needed an outlet to release her anger. Unfortunately, more often than not, that outlet was me.

. . . .

If it is true that beauty is in the eye of the beholder then it is also true we all play multiple roles in our lives and some are more or less attractive than others. This statement is especially apt for my mother who, as an amateur actress, became a different person on stage for each part she played. I recently discovered a black-and-white photo of her in a group shot of the cast and crew of a play that had just completed a successful run. The picture and the well wishes on the back side reveal a person I never knew—and yet, I was eight years old when the picture was taken.

My mother was then quite attractive. She smiles broadly, showing off a row of perfect white teeth. She has a round face with twinkling eyes and a small button nose. She is chubby, but not enough to stand out in a crowd.

More striking to me than the picture itself are some of the comments on the back side. From a couple of men in the crew: "Each performance is better than the last... And the first was excellent!!!" and "Dear Annette: I'll follow you wherever you go."

And from one of her younger colleagues, "If mothers could be chosen, I'd choose you. When I become a mother I want to be like you."

And from another, "To my dear 'mother,' I've enjoyed working with you on this play immensely."

I would have liked to have known this mother, even if it was just an act.

Albert

Albert Fried, born in 1931, grew up in the Williamsburg section of Brooklyn, a neighborhood populated mainly by first- and second-generation Jewish Americans from Eastern Europe. Williamsburg was undergoing a period of rapid growth and change during the 1930s and 1940s when Albert was growing up. The Jewish population of Williamsburg and Brooklyn in general had been sparse at the turn of the century, but this all changed with the opening of the Williamsburg Bridge in 1903. As described in an article from the Chosen Peoples Ministries website, "This structure, dubbed 'The Jew's Highway,' acted as a valve that channeled a vast influx of the overcrowded Jewish population of the Lower East Side into Brooklyn's Williamsburg section." In the late 1930s and 1940s, Jewish immigrants fleeing the Nazis also settled in Williamsburg. Many of these newcomers were Hasidic Jews, an Orthodox sect of Judaism. The Hasidic Jews opened numerous schools and synagogues and were very noticeable due to their all-black dress and the men's full beards. Their arrival had a major impact on the fabric of the neighborhood.

Economically, the people of Williamsburg, while not quite poor, still strived to make it into the middle class. Most households were headed by people who worked as unskilled laborers. The Bronx was about ten miles and a dream away.

Albert's parents were members of the lower working class. They had no more than grade-school educations and lived at the lower end of the income scale, but they always put food on the table and did not consider themselves to be poor.

Albert's family scrupulously observed Jewish law, but was not religious in a spiritual sense. They celebrated all of the Jewish holidays and conducted a short Sabbath prayer service every Friday night but rarely attended synagogue aside from Passover and the High Holy Days. They kept four sets of plates: dairy and non-dairy for Passover; dairy and non-dairy for the rest of the year. In short, they adhered to Jewish traditions, but not to the Jewish faith.

My parents followed Jewish tradition by naming me after my deceased grandfather. Our Jewish name, Israel, translates to "one who wrestles with God." Unfortunately my parents named me Ira, a common Americanization for boys with the Hebrew name Yisrael. If only they could have called me Isaac, or some other Jewish-sounding name that begins with an I, my life would have been so much easier.

Albert had only one sibling, Dorothy, who was three years older. Albert and Dorothy were very close as children and remained so throughout Albert's life. I recall the two of them calling each other every Sunday night, alternating who would make the call each week.

The defining event in Albert's childhood was the death of his father from eye cancer at the age of forty-one when Albert was ten years old. His father had been the sole breadwinner for the family, working as an unskilled laborer in a factory. His mother went to work as a seamstress to support the family. Albert and Dorothy never went hungry, but they knew their family had just enough to get by.

Albert was brilliant. I do not know his IQ, but I have no doubt it was not far from genius level. I didn't realize just how smart my father was until I was preparing for the GRE test, the equivalent of the SAT for liberal arts graduate programs, and was having difficulty with the logic section. This section had twenty-five questions and was to be completed within thirty minutes. I took practice test after practice test and could not get more than seventeen answers right. My father, seeing how frustrated I was, became curious and so decided to take the test himself. He completed the test in about twenty-five minutes, even with the distraction of two or three interruptions along the way. And despite never having seen the material before, he got twenty-two questions right, a score that would have put him in the ninety-ninth percentile for that portion of the test.

My father painted himself as a wise-guy street kid with a gang of friends who pulled off minor scams and pranks. He used to tell us that all his childhood friends were either dead or in jail. He wanted us to believe he was a ne'er-do-well who'd succeeded, despite growing up in a bad neighborhood, due to brains, pluck, and hard work.

As a young child, I believed his stories, but as I grew up I became increasingly skeptical. When I recently asked my Aunt Dorothy about his alleged exploits, she told me a story that described him in a way she felt was more typical. One evening, he and a few of his friends planned to run through the alley behind their houses later that night to knock over metal garbage pails set out to be picked up the next morning. Albert decided to go home before his gang committed their crime because he did not want to get in trouble for staying our too late. Dorothy said the worst thing he and his friends ever did was to let loose a bag of moths at the beginning of a movie.

My father liked to tell the story about how when he was in junior high he attended an end-of-year awards ceremony. Awards were given to the best student in each subject and, despite being a top student, he didn't receive any of them. And then, much to the chagrin of the school principal, who apparently knew Albert well for all the wrong reasons, Albert won the award for best overall student in his class.

Albert would later go on to high school at Brooklyn Tech, one of three elite public high schools in New York City at the time. The competition to get admitted into these schools was intense. After high school, Albert went to The Cooper Union to study engineering. The Cooper Union is a tuition-free college, located in lower Manhattan. It was, and still is, recognized for having one of the best engineering programs in the country. Competition to get in was even more intense than it was to get into

Brooklyn Tech. It was one of few options for people like Albert who couldn't afford to pay for college.

He continued to live at home, supported by his mother while attending college. Not until starting his first professional job, after graduating, did he have money for discretionary spending. Growing up as he did with so little money led him to be very frugal as an adult. He demonstrated this in ways that now seem a little strange, but amusing. For example, he always closely monitored the length of his Sunday evening calls with Dorothy to make sure they weren't too expensive, even after becoming a highly successful and well-compensated businessman. I also recall the time he ran out of gas on a long trip after he had passed gas station after gas station trying to find one with the lowest possible price.

As a child, I thought my father was cheap because he wouldn't buy me some of the things my friends had. It wasn't until much later that I appreciated that he was anything but cheap on the big items. Most notably, he paid the full cost of tuition and living expenses for college for my sisters and me. He also loaned me $5,000 for graduate school, which I am sure he never expected me to pay back—but I did.

Albert's mother also died at a relatively young age from cancer. I have only one extremely vague recollection of her from when I was not yet three years old, but from what I know of her, she must have been a remarkable woman. After Albert and Dorothy had grown up and left home, she continued to work the same long hours as she had before. She also continued to live the same Spartan lifestyle she had been forced to live while raising her children.

As a result, she was able to save a considerable portion of her earnings. She did this without telling anyone.

Albert and Dorothy knew their mother was putting some money aside, but had no idea how much. Seeing how hard she worked and how little she spent on herself, they urged her to take some time off from work and enjoy life a little. She refused. She continued to work and save money even after being diagnosed with cancer. By the time she died she had managed to save enough money to establish a college fund for each of my three cousins, Mandy, and me. (Edythe was born after our grandmother died.) She also left enough money for Dorothy to make a down payment on her first house and bequeathed a comparable amount to Albert.

Losing his father as a ten-year-old and seeing his mother die at a relatively young age after a lifetime of sacrifice had a profound impact on my father. Convinced he was not going to live beyond the age of fifty, he vowed that, unlike his mother, he would get as much enjoyment out of life as possible in the short time he had. Tragically, my father's premonition was right. He died of a massive heart attack a few days before his fifty-first birthday.

Wanting to maximize enjoyment may seem like a reasonable and perhaps even admirable way to live one's life. I personally do not have a problem with this attitude as long as one's pleasure does not come at the expense of others. There even exists an historical precedent of a moral philosophy built around the premise that one should seek to maximize pleasure. This philosophy, Epicureanism, had a wide following in ancient Rome before Christianity overtook it. Remnants of this philosophy exist today—the expressions "seize the day," "just do it," and "go for it" are more than just slogans.

My father had some great stories about how he succeeded by seizing an opportunity. The story that made the most lasting impression on me told of him taking a city-wide exam while in high school. He must have been an underclassman because as he told the tale, there was a set of questions that students in his grade were expected to answer, plus an additional set of questions that only the students in a higher grade were expected to answer. Because it was a timed standardized test, not many students in any grade finished before the allotted time and those who did simply put their pencils down and waited for the test to end for everyone else. My father completed the section of the test for his own grade well ahead of time. Then, instead of putting down his pencil, he decided to try answering some of the additional questions. It turned out that he got credit for the additional questions he answered correctly. As a result, despite not being one of the top students in his class, he got one of the highest scores for his grade in the entire city.

Looking at my father's philosophy of life through my own lens, I can see how it led him to behave in ways both very positive and very negative. On the positive side, I can remember him telling me over and over that if I saw an opportunity that would make a positive difference in my life, but seemed unattainable, I should go for it anyway. One of his favorite sayings was, "You already have a No; why not go for a Yes?" I have found myself frequently repeating this line when I give advice to my two boys, the people I managed at work, and the people I helped with my volunteer work.

My father's desire to enjoy life as much as possible had a negative side. The most significant was that it led him to behave in ways that were hurtful to people close to him. The person he hurt most was my mother. I do not know when it started, but I do know my father was seeing other women for a good portion of the time they were married. It is difficult to determine cause and effect. Did my father feel the need to seek the company of other women because my mother had become so unattractive both physically and as a person? How much did my father's treatment of my mother contribute to her anger and loss of self-esteem? It wasn't just the cheating on her that was cruel. He seemed to have a special talent for finding her most vulnerable spot and attacking her there when they argued. These are questions I have asked myself my entire adult life, but have never been able to answer.

Albert and Annette Together

Looking at their pictures from when they were young, I can see how there would be a physical attraction between the two. Albert was tall, lean, and handsome and Annette, while perhaps a little chubby by today's standards, had the looks of a Jayne Mansfield-type pin-up model. What I cannot tell from their pictures and is still a complete mystery to me is what else they saw in each other. I say that because, from my earliest recollections of them, when I was perhaps four or five years old, I cannot recall a single instance of them showing affection for each other. All I know about their courtship is that they met at one of the young Jewish adult singles camps that were popular at the time and that Albert must have really thought Annette

was special because he was willing to make the long sub-
way trek from Brooklyn to the Bronx and back again to
see her.

Both of my parents were strong-willed Type A person-
alities. Separately, they were successful in their respective
realms. Albert was a rising executive at General Electric,
one of the most respected companies of the day. Annette,
a stay-at-home wife and mother, was an officer of the local
chapter of B'nai B'rith, acted at a very highly regarded
local theater, painted, and had a reputation as an excellent
cook. Both were well-liked and respected by their peers as
leaders.

But together my parents were a perfect storm just waiting to happen. They fought constantly—never physically,
but they seemed to always be yelling at each other. The
silent treatment was in neither of their arsenals. I don't
remember what they were fighting about; I just remember
they were always fighting. Mandy, fourteen months older
than me, remembers them fighting mostly about seemingly insignificant issues, like whether they should go out to
dinner or stay home. Edythe, who is two and a half years
younger than me, also remembers them fighting constantly but does not remember any of the specifics.

An interest in politics is one of the few things my
parents shared. Both were huge Kennedy supporters and
were deeply affected by his assassination. One of my most
vivid early childhood memories is of them watching the
news and ceremonies on TV almost nonstop during the
days immediately following his assassination. I also have
vivid memories of my parents talking about how bad
Barry Goldwater, the far-right Republican presidential

candidate in 1964, would be for the country.

A few years later, when I was ten years old, I remember my parents watching the 1968 Democratic convention, transfixed. They were appalled by the demonstrations and infighting. I can clearly remember my father saying with disgust that we had just handed the election over to Nixon. Both of my parents continued to be interested in politics after 1968, but this was the last time I can remember them talking about politics as a shared interest.

Always keenly aware of his image, my father seemed at times to not only admire JFK, but to seek to emulate him. My father had the same haircut, was urbane and witty like JFK, and his favorite saying when one of my sisters or I complained we were being treated unfairly was the JFK quote, "Life is unfair." And in his professional life he was one of "the best and the brightest" at General Electric.

My mother, on the other hand, sometimes seemed to take on the persona of Maude, the TV character and nemesis of Archie Bunker, who loudly expressed her extremely liberal views. One incident that stands out in my mind occurred when I was about thirteen. A couple of young black women knocked on our door and asked for a donation to the Negro College Fund. My mother said she would gladly give a donation and she didn't care if they were purple with pink polka dots. I was so embarrassed, I had to hide.

Both of my parents faced difficult challenges, which helped to shape the people they became. My father reacted to the early death of his father and the sacrifices of his mother by pursuing his own enjoyment to the point where some of his behaviors can only be described as narcissistic. My mother reacted to the verbal abuse she suffered from her parents as a child and the indignities she suffered from being trapped in a terrible marriage by becoming increasingly insecure and angry.

CHAPTER 3
73 TOR COURT

I never lived in one place for more than five years at a time during my childhood. From the age of six to fourteen I moved five times, each time but the last into a bigger house. My family—father, mother, Edye (three and a half years younger than me), and Mandy (one year older)—became more dysfunctional with each change of address.

Pittsfield, with a population of about 60,000 in 1968, was and still is the largest city in Berkshire County, Massachusetts, or The Berkshires, as the county is more commonly known. Although surrounded by the natural beauty that made the Berkshires a popular tourist destination, Pittsfield itself was an industrial city with a predominantly blue collar population. Mostly white, the city also had a sizable black population, many of whom lived in "projects" located near the downtown area.

General Electric, by far Pittsfield's largest employer, had an outsized influence on the city and the people who lived there. According to one chronicler, GE had a "stranglehold on the local economy," which gave it a "lopsided influence on the city's development." Even the local arts were heavily dependent on GE's largess. As one of GE's top executives, my father undoubtedly was well-known as soon as he arrived.

During the period my family lived in Pittsfield, mid-

1968 through late-1972, the city and its residents enjoyed the last throes of a golden age. Blue-collar workers still earned enough to provide a comfortable middle-class life for their families, and professionals, especially those employed by GE, faired even better. Downtown Pittsfield, with its movie theaters, stores and restaurants, thrived. The terms "outsourcing" and "toxic waste site" were still unknown.

We moved from Lexington, Massachusetts, to Pittsfield two or three weeks before school started and, for the first several weeks, lived in a lakefront summer cottage. Onota Lake was the perfect recreational lake. About a mile wide and three miles long, it was big enough for sailing, but small enough to find calm waters for fishing and waterskiing. The owners of our temporary home allowed us to use their canoe and rowboat and my father put his beloved catamaran in the water. I took up fishing and quickly became addicted. Using the rowboat, I found a quiet spot on the far side of a short tunnel under a bridge that was just wide enough to for the boat to squeeze through. Here, it took no skill and very little effort to catch small sunfish.

One afternoon, after passing through the tunnel, I saw boy about my age standing on top of it. A skinny, funny-looking kid, he had short blond hair, big ears that stood out and a gawky way about him as he moved. We introduced ourselves to each other and quickly established we were next door neighbors. After a few more minutes of conversation I learned that, during the rest of the year, he lived only about a mile away from the house my family would soon occupy. Finally—I am not sure how the subject came up—he let me know he was Jewish, like me. Having gotten through the preliminaries, our conversation moved on to other topics. As we talked, we realized we liked many of the same things. We became fast friends.

School started a few days after I met Jerry. Uncomfortable being the new kid and concerned that people would pick on me as they had in Lexington, I was apprehensive. But at least I already had a friend. So I went school that first morning feeling nervous but hopeful I would get off to a good start.

My father dropped us off at Pomeroy Elementary and, with some help from Mandy, I found my fifth-grade classroom. A teacher, who I thought must be in her early nineties but later learned was in her fifties, greeted me, gave me a handout, and checked my name on an attendance sheet. Trying hard not to be noticed, I found a seat in the back of the room, where I sat fidgeting as I waiting for Mrs. W to speak.

Finally, after everyone had arrived and seated themselves, Mrs. W welcomed the class back to school. Next, she ran through a litany of things we'd better not do if we wanted to stay out of trouble. *This old lady is going to be one tough teacher,* I thought. She then explained that the class had been divided into three groups and we would each travel with our assigned group from class to class during three morning periods. My heart skipped a beat. From first grade on, my teachers had separated our classes for at least part of the day into groups—usually three—and everyone understood the groups were for the smart kids, the average kids, and what we thought were the dumb kids. Mrs. W directed us to the number next to our name on the first page of our handouts. I saw a "one" next to my name and breathed a sigh of relief. I knew I wouldn't be in the dumb group, so a one meant I had to be in the smart group. After that, I barely listened as Mrs. W prattled on about room assignments, our other teachers, and so on.

The bell rang, signaling us to move to our first period class. I hurried and once again found a seat in the back of the room. After everyone settled in our teacher took attendance. When she came to my name, she barked "Ira Fried. Where is she?" pronouncing my last name as it is spelled.

I shouted back, "I am Ira Fried and I am not a girl." I could feel my face get hot as I heard giggles from my classmates.

Caught off guard by my outburst the teacher then asked if Ira was a Jewish name. "Yes," I answered. This ten-second exchange validated all the reasons I had for hating my name.

I stewed all morning, until finally lunch time arrived. I followed Jerry to the cafeteria. After getting our food, we sat down at a table with some other kids he knew. His friends quizzed me about where I had moved from, where I lived now, whether I had any brothers or sisters, and so on. Although uncomfortable answering all these questions, I was pleased to have some of my new class-mates take an interest in me and relieved that none of them teased me about having a girl's name.

My family moved into our new house a few weeks after school started. Originally the driveway for a man-sion long since converted into a hospital, Tor Court was, according to my parents, the most prestigious street in Pittsfield. I recall my mother saying that during their first stint in Pittsfield she and my father would occasionally drive up and down Tor Court, dreaming that one day they might be able to live there. As we headed up the street toward our house, I started to wonder, "Why all the fuss?" Yes, the houses were big, but not that much bigger than the houses in our neighborhood in Lexington. My father drove slowly so he and my mother could take in the scene, as my sisters and I squirmed in our seats.

And then, there it was. On our left, behind a gravel, circular driveway stood a huge all-brick, H-shaped house. My father started down the driveway and for a few moments my attention turned to the sound of small stones crunching beneath the tires of our car. I still associate this sound with exclusivity and wealth.

We got out of the car and went in through the front door. We walked straight ahead to the kitchen and then turned left into the dining room/living room. Not normally one to get excited by a nice view, I had to stop and take notice after looking out the back window. Beyond a balcony that stretched from one end of the house to the other, and past a long sloping back yard, was a picture-postcard view of Onota Lake, with mountains in the background. I needed a better look so I went back to the kitchen, through the sliding glass doors and onto the balcony. From there I could see the back yard was flat for the first hundred feet or so, making it ideal for football. I then went back inside to explore the rest of the house.

I had grown accustomed to living in large houses, but this house was altogether different. Everything about it, from its size, to its design, to the property it sat on, exuded wealth.

Still on the main floor, at one end of the house, the master bedroom suite formed one of the vertical lines of the H. And at the other end, past the living room/dining room, another suite, with two large bedrooms separated by a bathroom, formed the other vertical line of the H.

The first thing I noticed when I got downstairs was how much cooler it was than upstairs. Then I noticed the size. With only three rooms in the finished portion, the lower level felt even bigger than the main level. Two of the rooms, a bedroom at least twice the size of my previous room, and a bathroom, were set off as a separate suite. The original owners of the house had designed this suite to serve as the maid's quarters. The other room, much too big to function only as a family room, most likely was intended by the original owners to serve as a party room—and indeed, my parents would put it to good use for that purpose. At one end of the room there was a fireplace and, at the other, a kitchen. My father arranged the TV, furniture, and a large area rug on the fireplace-end to make that space function as a family room. He put our ping pong table on the kitchen-end. My father and I could play ping pong while my mother and sisters watched TV, with little chance of interfering with each other.

Edye and Mandy each claimed a bedroom on the main floor, leaving me with the room on the lower floor. I didn't like this room. It made me shiver, partly from the cold, but also from the anxiety I felt at night, lying in my bed alone downstairs. My parents addressed the cold by giving me an electric blanket. But, too embarrassed, I never mentioned my anxiety. I stayed in this room for the first two years we lived in Pittsfield. Finally, at her behest, Mandy and I switched rooms. Almost fourteen by then, she understood the advantages of having a big room located far from her inattentive parents.

Only after seeing our house did I fully appreciate the fact that my family was rich. This realization gave rise to mixed feelings. I appreciated having all the things my family's income provided, but felt uncomfortable under the glare of the spotlight. Also, I felt a twinge of guilt—*have I become a spoiled rich kid?* I asked myself.

Our huge house, the views and the lakefront property told only part of the story. My father's status as one of the top executives at GE conveyed other, more subtle advantages as well. Adults frequently gave me favorable treatment for no good reason other than that I was my father's son. Mrs. W unofficially anointed me teacher's pet. Occasionally, as I slouched in my seat, trying to become invisible, she would use my father as an example of how a successful person behaves. Once, while making the case for the moral correctness of short hair, she asked me in front of the class how long my father wore his hair. This time, happy to answer, I replied—truthfully—my father had recently let his hair grow long enough to cover his ears. The class broke out in laughter. Much to my chagrin, Mrs. W continued to treat me as teacher's pet, despite this incident.

Jerry became my best friend. Despite his ungainliness, he loved sports as much as me. We had many other common interests as well: the Red Sox—he was almost as rabid about them as me—chess, ping pong, marbles, you name it. We could always find something to do.

Jerry and I did some pretty goofy things together. One time, both of us sat in the back row of the class room, Jerry in one corner, me in the other. We started making faces at each other. We continued for several minutes until finally I looked up and saw, much to my embarrassment, that the rest of the class was watching, barely able to contain their laughter. Mrs. W, having noticed us, had motioned to the rest of the class to quietly turn around and watch. It took a long time for Jerry and me to live that one down.

Jerry and I also suffered together through Hebrew School. Twice a week, we walked the mile and a half from Pomeroy Elementary School to the Jewish Community Center. To ease the pain of having to spend an hour and a half with Mr. or Mrs. Lebovich, who took turns teaching our class, we made a habit of stopping at Dunkin' Donuts on the way. There, I would get three cream-filled dough-nuts for 10 cents apiece.

Jerry and I joked that the Leboviches were certifiably crazy. Neither could control the class, despite sometimes taking extreme measures. Mrs. Lebovich, when angry, would stomp her high-heels near our toes, threatening in her heavily-accented English to crush them if we did not behave. Mr. Lebovich would alternate between yelling at us and muttering Jewish curses just loud enough to hear if we strained to listen. My favorite: "May you live like a chandelier. Hang by day and burn by night." At first, I behaved no worse than anyone else in the class, but over time I became increasingly disruptive. By the seventh grade, I was, more often than not, the person making Mr. or Mrs. Lebovich crazy. I made their lives miserable by never paying attention, making wisecracks, and interrupt-ing with deliberately inane questions. Usually, I got away with it, but eventually my behavior at Hebrew School led to severe consequences.

· · · · · · · · ·

It did not take long for my new classmates to start making fun of me, as they had in Lexington and even before then when we'd lived in Fairfield, Connecticut. I made a few friends at Pomeroy, but didn't consider them to be friends because they happily joined in when a group started to pick on me. But by then, having become accustomed to being the object of derision in school, I had developed a thicker skin, so it didn't bother me as much.

Nobody ever physically abused me during fifth or sixth grade, but for a few weeks during sixth grade, one kid, who I will call Bobby, regularly threatened to beat me up. In addition to these threats, he regularly hurled anti-Semitic slurs at me. I complained to my teacher and she told him to stop. He stopped for a few days but then started up again. Bobby came from a lower middle class family. His parents had not attended college and may not have graduated from high school. He had been assigned to the "dumb" group. Bobby's last name sounded a little like "bigot." One day, without having given it much thought, I called him Bobby Bigot. He asked me what bigot meant and I told him sneeringly to look it up. That stopped him in his tracks. Seeing the effect that had on him, I repeated, "Bobby Bigot, Bobby Bigot, Bobby Bigot!" Now with the upper hand, I called him Bobby Bigot every chance I had. He kept asking me what bigot meant and I kept telling him to figure it out himself.

This back and forth continued for a couple of days. Then, as we sat down next to each other at the beginning of the next school day, he looked at me with obvious pain and embarrassment and said "I'm not a bigot." He never bothered me again. Recalling this incident reminds me that the privileges I enjoyed extended beyond merely being rich and occasionally receiving special treatment by virtue of my father's status.

. . . .

I did not make friends easily. I had perhaps six or seven almost-friends with whom I ate lunch and hung out with during recess. But when school let out for summer, Jerry was the only friend I felt comfortable calling and asking to come over. My sisters and I usually went our own separate ways. So I also spent a lot of time by myself.

My parents had been at each other's throats for as long as I could remember, but now the fighting between them grew more intense. They fought more often, louder and with more intent to hurt each other. Both reacted by withdrawing—my father by increasing the lengths and frequency of his business trips, my mother by not participating in family activities. That summer my sisters and I—and my father when he was home—practically lived at the lake. But my mother went down there no more than two or three times all summer. Also, she stopped getting up in the morning to make us breakfast.

My relationship with her, strained since I was seven or eight years old, grew steadily worse. She yelled at me for the smallest offense—talking with food in my mouth, not doing a good job washing my face, not tucking my shirt in properly, and so on. And when she yelled, she was mean. She called me "an idiot's delight," a moron, and an imbecile, among other insults. Mandy recalls these outbursts as vicious slaps because each insult felt like a hard slap across the face.

My mother didn't have to yell to insult me. A fan of pop culture, she liked to talk about actors and the roles they played in different movies and TV shows. Occasionally, she couldn't identify the actor playing a specific role. Usually I remained silent, as I neither cared nor knew much about this topic. But one time, I thought I knew the answer and blurted it out. My mother turned on me saying, "You moron. How could anyone with a brain think he played that role? Idiot." And she went on to say, "You may have some book smarts but you have no common sense." My mother also loved to tell demeaning stories about me, like the time I hid under her bed after being scared by a loud thunder clap. I was five at the time.

A Random Act of Kindness

Sometimes, however, seemingly random acts of kindness come from the most unexpected sources. I was the recipient of such an act shortly after school had let out after fifth grade. My sisters and father went away for a few days, leaving just my mother and me at home. Each evening after dinner my mother went across the street to visit with a new friend she had made, leaving me alone until she came back well after dark. One evening, just before we were about to sit down for dinner, I heard a clap of distant thunder. I looked outside and saw the sky had darkened to a menacing mixture of black and gray, the wind bending some of the smaller tree branches close to the breaking point.

I hadn't seen lightning yet but it was obvious to me we were in for a violent storm. I told my mother that the storm was scaring me—I still hadn't completely outgrown my fear of thunderstorms. My mother told me not to worry—"everything will be okay." She then took an umbrella out of the front hall closet, gave me a scornful look, and went on her way.

Being alone at night in that big house was scary enough for me. Add to that my fear of thunderstorms, and I was genuinely frightened. I tried to be brave, but after about an hour I could not take it anymore.

I ran through the pouring rain to the house across the street and furiously rang the doorbell. The door opened and a woman I did not recognize appeared. I shouted past her to my mother that I was scared and I wanted her to come home. The woman who opened the door looked at me through friendly eyes and said, "Come on in." She sat me down at the table where my mother was still sitting and called for her high school-aged son, Paul, to bring some towels for me.

The woman asked Paul if he could hang out with me for a while. I was embarrassed but Paul put me at ease. He told me there was nothing wrong with getting scared. Then he talked to me about school, the Red Sox, fishing and whatever other topics came to mind, all the time making me feel like he was genuinely glad to have my company.

The next day I got a call. It was Paul. He wanted to know if I would like to go fishing with him the next morning. Of course, I said yes. For the rest of the day I couldn't stop telling my mother how honored I was that someone in high school would actually want to go fishing with me.

The following morning we put the boat in the water before 6 a.m. and continued fishing until about noon. Then we had peanut butter and jelly sandwiches that his mother had made for us. I had a terrific time. I will never forget Paul for his kindness.

As I reflect on this incident, I wonder if I also owe my mother a debt of gratitude. Did she ask Paul to take me fishing? Did his mother ask him? Or did he decide on his own? I will never know. But I would like to hold out the possibility that at least this one time my mother did something incredibly nice for me.

CHAPTER 4
CROSBY JUNIOR HIGH

Several times larger than Pomeroy Elementary School, Crosby Junior High intimidated me at first. No longer a ruler of the playground as a sixth grader in elementary school, I was now a seventh-grader in a seventh through ninth grade school. The first day, while walking through the crowded hallway to one of my classes, I heard a boy yell out "grab a tit" as he passed by some girls. No one ever talked that way in elementary school! Just finding the right room was a challenge for the first few days. I felt like I was in over my head.By the end of the first week, however, I had become accustomed to the new routine and began to feel more comfortable.

Then the first real change hit. Girls! They became my primary focus. During sixth grade I had a crush on a girl, but our relationship never went beyond me stealing glances at her and her occasionally catching me in the act. At Crosby Junior High we took relationships between boys and girls to a whole new level: we exchanged secret notes about who liked who. Some of the more popular boys would not have considered exchanging notes with girls—they had their strong, tough images to protect.

The object of my affection, Kate, had light brown hair down to her shoulders, big brown eyes and an inviting smile. I enjoyed bantering with her and also liked that she was smart. I needed to find out if she had similar feelings for me. And if it took passing notes around to find out, then so be it.

For a short while I became very close friends with Bill, an acquaintance from elementary school. Bill, widely regarded as the smartest kid in the seventh grade class, looked about two years younger than the rest of us. People gave him grudging respect for being so smart but also considered him to be the ultimate nerd. Bill had a crush on Carol, a very pretty girl who appeared to be the leader among her group of friends. Carol could be nice to boys she or one of her friends liked, but had very little time for someone she considered to be below her in the social pecking order. Despite Bill's numerous attempts to get her attention, she barely acknowledged his existence. She was way out of Bill's league.

Bill and I talked every chance we got about Kate and Carol. On days I didn't have Hebrew school I went to his house—about ten minutes away by bike—where we talked strategy about how and when to ask them out, even though we didn't know what "going out" with a girl meant.

My friendship with Bill ended abruptly not much longer than a month after it began. Carol invited me to a "boy-girl" party but did not invite Bill. I merited an invitation because Carol's friend, Kate—yes, the same Kate—liked me. I pleaded with Carol to invite Bill, but she refused. So I did what any love-struck twelve-year-old boy would do: I abandoned Bill and went to the party without him.

I arrived a little late, as planned. Carol welcomed me, took my jacket, and led me to the basement, where the dim lighting and blaring music announced a party was being held. Before we reached the last step Carol stopped me and whispered in my ear that Kate had arrived earlier and was waiting for me. Still whispering in a barely audible voice, Carol instructed me to go over to Kate and ask her to dance. With these words Carol eliminated any residual doubts I had about why I had been invited to the party.

I helped myself to a cup of punch and ambled over to where the other boys were standing. I didn't know any of them well but that didn't matter. I had come to the party for only one purpose: Kate. Then I saw her, radiant in a brown pant suit. She was looking at me! I strode over to her, trying my best to look confident and relaxed while praying I did not trip and fall. I made it to her, without incident, and shouted over the din of the music, "Hi Kate. Would you like to dance with me?"

I couldn't hear her response but her broad smile told me she had answered, "Yes."

After a few fast-dance songs, someone put The Jackson Five's "I'll Be There" on the record player. I asked Kate if she wanted to keep dancing and she said yes with a smile that made my legs wobble. I put my arms around her waist and then she pulled me toward her so that our bodies were pressed against each other. Overcome with a combination of love and lust, I thought to myself, *If there is a heaven, this must be it.* I knew then in my love-addled brain that, as the chorus of the song went, I would be there for Kate whenever she needed me.

By the end of the party Kate and I had slow-danced four more times, each time as wonderful as the first. But we never went to one of the dark corners of the base-ment, where several other couples had gone to make out.

I wanted to tell Kate how I felt about her but I couldn't find the right words and I didn't want to risk breaking the mood by trying to kiss her at the wrong time or in the wrong way.

The party ended abruptly for me when my father came to pick me up. I said to Kate, "My dad's here. Gotta go. I had a great time. See ya on Monday."

A wave of frustration and self-loathing washed over me as Kate replied with disappointment and hurt. "Yeah, I had a good time too. See ya on Monday."

As we started the drive home, my father asked if I had a good time. I told him I had. Then he asked who I had been talking to when he picked me up. I said, "A friend," and we drove the rest of the way home in silence.

Having satisfied my father, my thoughts returned to Kate. I resolved to ask her on Monday morning if she would "go out with me." But I couldn't summon the courage to do it. Every time I thought I was ready I found another excuse to wait. At the end of the week, frustrated and angry with myself, I knew I had missed my opportunity. And so ended my first attempt at romance....

· · · · · · · · ·

Exacerbating my pain and frustration, my mother saw Carol's party as a good reason to resume her on-and-off questioning about girls. Any mention of the opposite sex directed my way deeply embarrassed me. My father seemed to understand and never pushed too hard. But I think my mother enjoyed watching my discomfort as she pursued this line of questioning.

During breakfast the next morning my mother asked whether I had fun at the party. I muttered "Yes," without saying another word. Then my mother asked whether I met someone special there. This time I replied with an emphatic "No." With my father there, my mother stopped her interrogation.

A couple of weeks later, when my father was away on business, my mother started again where she had left off. She asked me whether I was afraid of girls. "No," I replied to her with false bravado. "I can take any girl in my class."

"You know that's not what I meant," she persisted, but I refused to say anything else. Then she released the heavy bombs she had been storing. She asked, "Do you like girls?"

Feeling tension rise throughout my body, I said, "I don't know. I guess so."

But my mother, having cornered her quarry, persisted. "Any particular girl?" she asked.

I shouted back, "No," but she continued malevolently.

"Would you like me to get you *Playboy Magazine?*"

By then, feeling a mixture of intense rage and embarrassment, I said nothing. Then my mother, ever the supportive parent, asked if perhaps I would prefer a magazine with pictures of men. I stormed out of the room crying, ending the inquisition.

Going Downhill

Seventh grade marked the beginning of a steep decline in my academic performance. As I became more comfortable at Crosby, I gradually took on the role of class clown.

I hadn't consciously aspired to this position. I probably made a few wisecracks and got some reassuring laughs. Then, enjoying the positive feedback, made a few more, got some more laughs and so on. At first, even my teachers appreciated my humor. But I didn't know when to stop. I relished the attention and the more I got, the more I needed. Before long, my teachers, no longer amused by my frequent interruptions, started telling me to stop. I still respected authority enough in seventh grade for this intervention to contain my addiction, but in eighth grade it spun out of control.

The junior high bullying started about midway through seventh grade. Robert, a kid in my home room who lived in the projects, was the first to bully me. Constantly shoving and challenging me to fight him, he was relentless. I don't know why he picked me—perhaps he found out where I lived and resented me for it. But I can see why he kept it up once he started. I never fought back—I just cowered each time he taunted me. I was the perfect victim. Afraid of what he would do if I did fight back, I let him continue to shove and taunt me. Nobody ever said anything to me about it, but everyone in the class, including the teacher, had to have been aware of what was going on.

One day I was walking home from school with Mark, an acquaintance with whom I got along well. Suddenly, Frank, another acquaintance, snuck up on us and tried to jump me from behind. Hearing him just in time, I bent over at the moment he would have landed on me. I flipped him, letting his momentum do most of the work, and he landed in a heap at my feet. We all broke out laughing. I had just pulled off a pretty impressive move. Mark and I razzed Frank as he got up. But as we started walking,

Frank asked—without intending any malice—why I never did that to Robert. Frank had unintentionally revealed me as being capable of defending myself against Robert. I had no reason not to fight back other than cowardice. I doubt Mark or Frank told anyone else about the incident, but it stuck with me.

In my interactions with Robert, discretion may actually have been the better part of valor. A few weeks later he started in on someone else. This kid had a reputation as someone who most people would not want to mess with. He fought back. Robert knocked the kid unconscious and started jumping on him until a teacher finally intervened. The kid, who had to be taken away in an ambulance, suffered a concussion and two broken ribs. I never saw Robert again.

I was relieved to be rid of Robert but by then the damage was done. I had established a reputation as an easy mark for bullies. A succession of people took advantage. I always had an excuse for not fighting back: I had a sprained neck, my arm still hurt from the flu shot I had just received, I didn't see how fighting proved anything, and on and on. Each time this happened, I lost a little more respect from my peers and myself.

My Grand Theory

At the end of seventh grade, with too much time on my hands, I developed my "Grand Theory of Why People Get Picked On." Every group of people, whether large or small, I reasoned, needs a pariah. Groups define themselves not only by who they are and what they believe, but also by what they are not. People who behave or look different function as sign posts for the majority, helping them to define what they are not. The Jews played this role in Nazi Germany. Blacks played it in the American South. Merely recognizing people who are different is not enough, though. By attacking people who are different, the majority group defines itself more clearly and demonstrates its superiority.

My "Grand Theory" helped me cope just a little better by providing an explanation for why every group needs a pariah. But it didn't shed any light on why that pariah always seemed to be me. I knew my inability to stand up to bullies contributed. I also suspected my behavior in class had an impact. But I also knew there was more to it than that. After all, people had been picking on me since second grade, long before I started acting out in class. Had I been more aware of how people perceived me I might also have realized I was the antithesis of cool. I shared notes with girls. I wore the ill-fitting, sometimes outrageous, clothes my mother chose for me. And I lacked the tough, apathetic exterior most boys my age presented, freely sharing my thoughts and emotions.

A Downward Spiral

Having become bored spending so much time by myself trying to solve the riddles of the universe, I welcomed the beginning of the new school year. And for the first two or three weeks, not yet knowing what my teachers would tolerate, I behaved well. Luckily, I had a couple of outstanding teachers that year whom I held in high esteem. For them, my conduct was exemplary. For example, my algebra teacher, Mr. M, whose very presence commanded respect, simply would not have tolerated poor behavior. In his class I paid attention, completed my assignments on time, and refrained from making any inappropriate comments—and I performed well. I also had a lot of respect for my English teacher. Tough, but fair, she set the bar high for us. I worked hard in her class, too, and earned a B for the first two quarters' grade, narrowly missing an A both times.

But these two classes were the exceptions. Starved for attention, I resumed playing the role of class clown in the rest. I became increasingly disruptive. As my teachers threatened me with all manner of punishment, my classmates egged me on. Even if my jokes were not always funny, they enjoyed the spectacle of my confrontations with the teachers. They gave me the attention fix I needed, so I continued with this behavior, not caring about the consequences.

I was especially hard on my history teacher. She lacked command of the class, in large part due to the commotion I created. I will always regret the time when, in response to someone asking whether she was married, I shouted out, "No. She's too ugly." As I spoke our eyes locked. I could see as soon as the words came out of my mouth how hurtful they were to her. I felt a knot in my stomach. I knew I should go up to her after class and apologize but I couldn't face her. I never did apologize.

I behaved even worse in Hebrew School. And there I suffered the consequences sooner. The Leboviches, thoroughly fed up with my antics, finally convinced the school to expel me. At first I was happy to hear the news—No more Hebrew School! Unfortunately, my father had a somewhat different perspective. Furious with me and concerned I would not get a proper Jewish education, he went to the school and somehow convinced them to let me rejoin my class. When he got home he grounded me and banned me from watching TV for two weeks. He also threatened to extend this punishment indefinitely if he heard "so much as a peep" about me misbehaving again.

Meanwhile, my performance continued its downward trajectory at Crosby. My English teacher went on an extended family leave at the end of second quarter. I showed absolutely no respect for her substitute, constantly interrupting her and putting very little effort into my work. She generously gave me a C for my third quarter grade.

I did even worse in the non-academic subjects. Having little aptitude for or interest in music and art, I rarely paid attention in these classes. I frequently asked questions and made inappropriate comments purposely to distract my teachers—and, of course, to get attention. But I made at least a pretense of doing my work and did well on the tests so I managed to get a C in both of these classes as well.

My substitute English teacher's generosity and the low standards in art and music classes left me with the impression I could get away with anything. So in the fourth quarter I took my behavior up another notch. I added to my repertoire refusing to participate constructively in any classroom discussions and skipping assignments. I stopped altogether doing any work in music and art.

At the end of the last day of school our home room teachers gave us our final report cards. I knew my fourth quarter grades would be bad but I hoped they would at least be good enough to keep me out of trouble. Fortunately I was seated when I opened my report card because otherwise I might have collapsed. I looked in disbelief at the D in the fourth quarter box for English and the Fs in the boxes for music and art. In addition to the letter grade, we received a 1, 2, or 3 for effort and behavior, with 1 being the best. Teachers rarely gave out 3s, but I got a 3 in all three classes. With the exception of a B in Mr. M's algebra class, my report card was strewn with Cs, Ds and Fs. The final bell rang and everyone got up to leave. I stayed seated at my desk, too stunned to move.

After a few minutes of sitting in the classroom by myself, my home room teacher tapped me on the shoulder and told me it was time to go home. With unsteady legs I got up and left.

As I walked home I considered my options: should I try to convince my father I didn't have the report card? No, he would find out anyway and lying would only make him angrier. Should I run away from home? But where would I go? I had no way out. I had to give the report card to him.

My father had injured his back in a car accident a few months earlier and often, after a full day of sitting at his desk, it hurt. On the bad days he would lie in bed after dinner. Fortunately for me, this was one of those days. I knew I could get away if he became enraged, as I expected he would after seeing my report card. I knocked on the door to his room, he told me to come in and I entered, my legs trembling so badly I could barely walk. Noticing, he asked me what was wrong. I told him in a barely audible voice that I had my report card and then, as I pulled it out of my pocket, I stammered out the words, "It's probably not quite as good as you're expecting."

I handed it to him gingerly and waited for him to

erupt. But he didn't. He looked at me calmly and said, "This is unacceptable. I will let you know when I am ready how you will be punished." The next day he told me I would lose all lake privileges for four weeks. Then he really surprised me. He laughed and said, "Well I'm glad to see you got a 3 for effort in the classes you failed. I would be worried if you had tried and then got an F." Still too nervous to laugh with him, I waited for him to tell me I could leave and then slinked out of the room. Incidentally, that was the first time I can recall him exhibiting a trait I now realize I inherited from him. He could become enraged by relatively small annoyances—like getting caught in a traffic jam. But he was always the picture of calm when something big happened.

And it's No Better at Home

While my performance at school had plummeted, my family life had also continued its downward spiral. My father, having significantly increased his business travel, was away almost as much as he was home. And when he was home, he and my mother fought constantly. Usually, the fighting started within an hour or two of his arrival. My mother seemed almost to look forward to his return so she could start yelling at him. My mother stepped up her attacks on me, especially when my father was not home. I started to fight back and the yelling between the two of us soon became another constant of life at 73 Tor Court.

By then, my mother had all but abdicated her responsibilities as a parent. She still made dinner and shopped for us, but that was about it. She didn't take an interest in our friends. She didn't seem to care where we went or how long we stayed out—Mandy regularly came home past eleven on school nights and my mother never questioned her about it. She didn't even ask to see our report cards anymore.

Despite the financial and social privileges we enjoyed living on Tor Court, happiness eluded us all. Edythe, only ten at the time, recalls thinking, "Now, I am on my own." I remember feeling much the same way.

John and his Friends

So many times, when I needed it most, someone came into my life and made a huge positive difference for me. My neighbor Paul, who took me fishing, was the first. John was the second. Near the end of summer between seventh and eighth grade he told me his family would be moving next door to us. Although I didn't know them well, John and his brother David both seemed like decent enough guys, so I was excited to have them as neighbors.

John, a garrulous, outgoing person, was hard not to like. Always upbeat, nothing seemed to bother him. But beneath his friendly, devil-may-care exterior, he also had a serious, thoughtful side. I cannot recall whether I told him about my "Grand Theory" but I am sure he would have understood it if I did. He became my best friend, even if I was not his.

John went to Catholic school, so he didn't see how I acted in class or how my classmates treated me. But he had several friends at Crosby, including his best friend, Matt, so he, no doubt, knew how unpopular I was. None of that seemed to bother him, though. He seemed to get a kick out of, and perhaps even found endearing, some of the same qualities that prompted most other guys to tease and taunt me: my guilelessness, gullibility, even my clueless-ness about clothes.

I vividly recall the time I was doing yard work and John came over to me convulsing in laughter. I couldn't figure out why he was laughing so hard. At first I thought he might be laughing because I was stuck working in the yard on such a beautiful day. But he was laughing much too hard for that. Finally, he pointed to my legs and, after another spasm of laughter, managed to spit out the words: "You can't wear those pants in public." I stood there wearing red, white, and blue bellbottoms my mother had bought for me, oblivious as to how ridiculous they made me look. But whereas most guys would have exulted at the opportunity to mock me and invite others to join him, John—after recovering from his laughter—just said, "Seriously man, you need to get rid of those pants." I never heard about that incident from John or anyone else again.

I think John may also have appreciated that, around me, he could shed the veneer of apathy and toughness most boys our age wore. He could admit he liked, and even start dancing to, a pop song—long since forgotten—that ranked just a notch above my yard work attire on the coolness scale. He could also safely talk with me about more serious top-ics, like God and religion, our families, the most important qualities—in addition to physical attractiveness—to look for in a girlfriend, and anything else that mattered. Dis-cussions such as these required a modicum of introspection and intellectual curiosity, traits that were anathema to the image most boys our age wanted to project. I wore them, like my emotions, on my sleeve.

John hung out with a group of three and sometimes four guys; all but one went to Crosby. Of all of them, Matt, who had also gone to Pomeroy, gave me the hardest time. They all knew me well and none of them had the least bit of interest in hanging out with someone as dorky as me. But John regularly invited, even encouraged, me to join him when he got together with them. I usually accepted John's invitation and as a result became a part of this group.

Matt and the others may have allowed me to join their group, but they made it crystal clear I did not belong. With one notable exception—when Matt obtained a pack of firecrackers and, one at a time, lit them and tossed them in my direction, barely missing me a few times as they exploded—John's friends never abused me physically. But they mocked me constantly–about how little I knew about music, my misguided attempts at humor, the seriousness with which I took most conversations, and even occasionally, the fact that I was Jewish. But having long since become accustomed to this type of treatment, it didn't bother me most of the time. That was my world and I had learned to live in it. I actually enjoyed hanging out with John's friends when they were not picking on me. I preferred being an outcast in this group to not being in any group at all.

Despite their obvious distain for me, Matt and the others rarely excluded me. I think they may subconsciously have wanted me in their group because they enjoyed having someone to laugh at. Per my Grand Theory, their group, like every other, needed a pariah. We had reached a point of equilibrium, where both parties gave up something and got something in return. But even the most stable systems don't usually stay in equilibrium. Some outside force inevitably upsets the balance.

The outside force in this instance was one of John's friend's discovery of the progressive rock group, Yes. We spent a lot of time listening to music and held strong opinions about what was good and what was not. Everyone agreed the music played on AM stations was "bubble gum" pop intended for "teeny boppers" and other un-worthies. With album-rock FM still in its infancy and largely unknown to most kids our age, current knowledge of serious rock conveyed a certain degree of coolness. Considering me the epitome of un-coolness, John's friends only grudgingly allowed me to participate when they listened to music.

Then one of John's friends discovered Yes and played their first album for us. We listened to the record, transfixed. We had never heard anything that sounded like Yes before—the album blew us away. But then, seeing my excitement—which, given my nature, I probably expressed more vigorously than anyone else—they turned on me. A discovery like this was reserved for the coolest of the cool and having someone as uncool as me in the room took away from a special moment. They allowed me to stay only at John's insistence.

About a week later, I announced I had bought the Yes album. Matt took the group's line of thinking regarding music to its logical extreme. He broke into my room and stole the record. Breaking in was not hard because I had switched rooms with Mandy by then and my room had a door to our balcony, which until then I had left unlocked.

I soon realized the album was missing and, in my last desperate attempt to find it, I asked John's friends if any of them had seen it. About a week later—probably at John's behest—Matt returned it. He explained he had taken it because I didn't deserve to listen to anything as good as Yes. Hurt by what Matt had done but happy to have my album back, I continued to hang out with John and his friends.

Second Attempt at Romance

If baseball was the most popular sport when we lived in Lexington, skiing was the sport of choice in Pittsfield. We had our own little ski resort right in town. With a vertical rise of only 600 feet, Bousquet Mountain was tiny compared to the Vermont resorts. But within twenty minutes of leaving our house, we could be in the lodge putting on our boots. Convenient and affordable, skiing at Bousquet was a popular winter activity for families in Pittsfield. Many of the kids I knew from school skied there regularly. Frequently, several of us would find each other there and end up skiing or sometimes just hanging out in the lodge together. For thirteen-year-old kids, Bousquet was as much a place to socialize as it was a place to ski.

A couple of days before Christmas break, Kate let me know—through the usual channels, using Carol as the go-between—that she still liked me. I didn't have to reply. Kate could tell by the way I started fidgeting in my seat and tripping over my words when I tried to talk to her that I still liked her too. She asked me whether I planned to do any skiing over the break. I said yes, but couldn't think of anything else to say. I had known Kate for almost a year and a half by then and, with the exception of three or four awkward weeks after the boy-girl party in the seventh grade, I had always found it easy to talk with her. I didn't realize it at the time, but Kate had become a friend who happened to be a girl. But the moment she became a potential girlfriend everything changed. Along with the rush of excitement, I could feel my whole body get tense whenever I got near her. My brain seemed to go into a deep freeze as I struggled to find the right words to say. I felt awkward and gangly, as if my arms and legs had suddenly become too big to fit my body.

John and I had already made plans to ski during the break. His mother had agreed to take us to Bousquet each morning and my father, who hoped to take time off to ski at least a few afternoons that week, agreed to take us home. On the way to Bousquet the day after Christmas, John's mother asked me a question but, lost in thought, I didn't reply. I was thinking about Kate. *What should I say if I see her? Should I just come right out with it and ask her to ski with me? No, that won't sound right. I should make some small talk first. But what should I say? How did I get myself into this mess anyway?*

Then I heard John's mother ask: "Ira, are you okay?"

After his mother dropped us off, John asked what was wrong with me. Then I made my first big mistake. I told John about Kate. A couple of hours later I made my second big mistake. Seeing Kate on the chair lift after we stopped on the slope underneath to catch our breath, I pointed her out to him. From that point on, John was relentless. At the end of the day he spotted her taking off her skis. He called out her name and started walking toward her while I stood frozen like a statue. Not recognizing the voice, Kate looked up. John called out her name again and proceeded toward her. By then, realizing my only other option was to run and hide, I quickly caught up to him. A few moments later, Kate noticed me walking toward her with John. The three of us, plus a friend Kate had been skiing with, talked for a few minutes before John and Kate's friend found excuses to go someplace else. Kate and I then talked for a few more minutes, but the best I could do was ask her whether she planned to go skiing the next day. She said yes.

I said, "Great. I hope to see you tomorrow," and headed into the lodge, where John waited for me. John, all over me for not arranging a time to meet Kate, told me in no uncertain terms I would ask her to ski with me the next day.

The next day, as we prepared to hit the slopes again following a brief lunch break, John saw Kate outside standing next to her friend. He practically pushed me out the door of the lodge, demanding I ask her to ski with me. Gathering up my courage, I walked up to her and, after somehow managing to make small talk for a couple of minutes, asked her. Kate said yes and her friend, no doubt well-prepped by Kate, graciously went off to ski with someone else.

Skiing was the perfect activity for a date. We had no choice but to sit right next to each other on the chair lift and the ride up the mountain provided plenty of alone time to talk and possibly even make out. I thought I had gone to heaven as Kate and I rode up the first time. But then I spotted my father skiing below us and everything went awry. Still too uncomfortable talking about girls with him to let him know I had a girlfriend, I became paranoid he would see Kate and me together. From that moment on, all I could talk about with Kate was how I didn't want my father to see us. I skied fast, making her hurry to keep up with me. Wondering what was wrong with me, she asked with exasperation whether I would get in trouble if my father saw us. I said no, but could not explain any further. It must have been an awful experience for Kate. After stopping to take a break, we agreed not to ski with each other for the rest of the day. I ended up skiing with my father. He asked me who I had been skiing with and I said, "Just a friend." And so ended my second attempt at romance.

CHAPTER 5
GOD, RELIGION AND DIVORCE

Visit to the Holy Land

Shortly after school ended, my family took a trip to Israel. I considered myself incredibly lucky to go on this trip. In 1972, air travel had not yet become commonplace, as it is today. Most of my classmates had never been on a plane, much less flown to a country halfway around the world. Also, years of indoctrination had taught me that Israel was a special place every Jew should visit at least once in his life—"Next year in Jerusalem" was a common refrain during Passover Seders.

I vividly recall many of the sites we visited. I remember floating on the Dead Sea. The next day we climbed to the top of Masada, where the Jews fought the Romans until, their numbers dwindling, they made a suicide pact so none would remain when the Romans finally took over. Jerusalem, many of its buildings pock-marked from bullets fired during the 1967 Six Day War, was both interesting and disquieting—watching my father barter with the merchants, many of whom only five years earlier had been firing those bullets, gave me a strange, slightly uncomfortable feeling. Especially memorable for me was our visit to the Temple Mount and Wailing Wall, considered the holiest of holy places for Jews. Israel had returned The Wall, for many the symbol of the Jewish diaspora, to Jewish control after two thousand years in foreign hands. As

I observed people praying at The Wall, the emotion they expressed was palpable.

Nevertheless, the trip was a wretched experience for me and the rest of the Fried family. My father meticulously planned every stop. We spent the first week in the desert, riding from site to site in a car without air conditioning. The daytime temperature exceeded 100 degrees that entire week. By the middle of the week, my mother developed a severe sunburn on the arm she had rested on the window during our drive through the desert. The sites, mostly excavations, ruins, and ancient settlements, had all begun to look alike to my sisters and me. But no matter how hot and tired we were, or how much pain my mother felt, my father insisted on stopping at every site on his itinerary. By the end of that first week we were all in a terrible mood.

We spent the next week in Jerusalem. One day my father and sisters went on a horseback riding excursion. Afraid of riding horses, I elected to stay back at the hotel with my mother. That morning at breakfast she badgered me nonstop about my table manners. "You have crumbs on your face," she bellowed. "Don't pick up the next piece of food until you've swallowed what's in your mouth. Take smaller bites." My temper rising, I asked her in a voice several decibels above normal why she had to pick on me. She replied, her voice getting louder, "You moron, how are you going to amount to anything if you can't even eat right? You eat like a pig."

No longer able to contain my anger, I yelled back, "Just leave me alone—I don't need to learn all this crap."

Her face twisted in rage, my mother slapped me hard across the face. I sat at the table crying for a few minutes and then ran back to the room. I cried not from the physical pain of the slap, but from the anger and shame I felt from it. The worst moment of the trip for me came the next morning at breakfast when our waiter asked me in his broken English, loudly enough for the people at the next table to hear, "You cry yesterday?"

We spent the last week of our trip at a couple of different kibbutzes. On the way, we drove through the Golan Heights, territory that Israel had captured from Syria during the Six Day War. Even for someone who knew almost nothing about military strategy, the importance of the Heights was readily apparent. From the vantage point of a former Syrian pill box—a long, narrow concrete structure built into the hill, with narrow slits for shooting the only openings in the front—we could see how easily the Syrians were able to shoot at the people working at the kibbutzes in the valley below.

By the time we finished exploring the pill box, the sun had begun to go down. Seeing that, I felt a chill run down my spine. I grabbed the guide book and turned to the page on the Golan Heights. The book confirmed my worst fears. "Warning!" it said. "Do not travel in the Golan Heights past dusk." But to no avail. My father, wanting to see more, drove further into the Heights, as the rest of us grew increasingly nervous. Finally, feeling curious, he drove past a No Entry sign and continued down a dirt road. A few hundred yards later, a man we immediately identified as an Arab by his traditional clothing stepped into the road in front of us waving his arms furiously. I thought he was going to kill us. But he was trying to help. Aware we were in a buffer zone headed toward the Syrian border, he was signaling us to turn around. My father turned the car around and started heading out of the Heights. For the next half hour, until we reached the valley floor, all of us except my father felt unbridled fear.

Early Musings on Religion

I thought a lot about God and religion during the time I lived in Pittsfield—more so than most kids my age. Most of what I thought was pretty negative. The Saturday morning Sabbath services got me started thinking this way. They lasted easily two and a half hours and were conducted primarily in Hebrew, a language few people in the congregation understood. I was bored senseless during these services. I had to think of something to avoid going crazy. I chose to think about all the things I didn't like about religion.

My father's hypocrisy also had an impact. On Saturday mornings, he would drop my sisters and me off at synagogue and then go to work rather than joining us. Yet on Yom Kippur he was always the most pious man in the congregation. Services went on all day long and my father attended for almost the entire day. He criticized my mother, sisters, and me for not spending more than the several hours we already spent at services. If my father was such a good Jew, I wondered, why did he practice his religion only one day a year?

But I think Hebrew School, especially the afternoon classes, had the greatest impact. I disliked these classes not only because I found them boring, but more importantly because I thought the material we covered had no relevance to me. We learned to read Hebrew—not to understand the language, but to learn how to properly enunciate Hebrew text. We learned a little vocabulary—perhaps enough to speak like a native two-year-old by the time I was thirteen—and we discussed each of the Jewish holidays as they came up on the calendar.

The Sunday classes were only slightly better. We spent most of our time learning the stories of the Bible—which our teachers presented as being literally true. We also learned about the history of the Jewish people from ancient times up to and including the Holocaust. But most importantly, we learned that the Jews were God's Chosen People.

Every once in a rare while we were asked to do an exercise that required us to think. The one I remember best was assigned by a substitute teacher when I was in fifth or sixth grade. The teacher asked us to describe God. I answered that God was an old man, dressed well, and that God was love. The second half of my answer was based on a billboard I had recently seen. It merited a C+, one of the highest grades in the class for that exercise. At that young age, I had already become cynical about religion.

By the time I reached twelve, I doubted most of what I had learned in Hebrew School. I no longer believed any of the stories from the Bible. The story of Noah and his ark seemed especially far-fetched to me. It would be impossible to build a boat large enough to fit a male and a female animal of each species. Also, how were two animals of each species chosen for the ark? What did they eat during their journey? Did some of the animals eat others, leaving fewer of Noah's guests at the end of the journey than at the beginning?

It also didn't make sense to me that God would single out Jews as The Chosen People. Why would God choose us over everyone else? By the same token, it didn't make sense to me that Catholicism could be the One True Church or any other religion could somehow be superior to the rest in the eyes of God. The Holocaust, still fresh in the minds of people my parents' age when I was growing up, was often used as an example of how we were The Chosen People. The Leboviches, Holocaust survivors themselves, taught that we had been chosen by God to suffer in the Holocaust and our suffering reaffirmed our status as the Chosen People. But I believed the Holocaust had nothing to do with God. In my mind the Jews were just the unfortunate victims of a vicious, hateful regime.

The more I thought about religion, the more certain I became that organized religions were bad for society. In my mind, they were just a way of separating people into different groups that more often than not hated each other because of their differences. By the time I was thirteen, my history classes in school had covered the beginning of Christianity through the present day. Too many wars had been fought over religion and too many people had been oppressed for holding religious beliefs that were different from those of the dominant religion, I reasoned, for organized religion to possibly be a good thing.

I still believed in God's existence. *Who else but a God could have created the world?* I reasoned. But I didn't have any idea of what God was really like. Was he really loving, all-knowing and all-powerful, as I had learned in Hebrew School? Was he really watching over me and, if so, was he really ready to punish me if I did something wrong? If God is loving, all-knowing and all-powerful, why did he let the Holocaust happen?

I also still believed in heaven and hell but I did not believe that hell was fire and brimstone. Instead, I believed hell was more like an episode of "The Twilight Zone" I had seen, where a hippie is doomed to watch a staid middle-aged couple show their vacation slides for eternity. Hell is different for each person. For some reason, I didn't give nearly as much thought to heaven.

Like every boy in even mildly observant Jewish families, I was expected to be Bar Mitzvah'd shortly after my thirteenth birthday. In the Jewish faith, a Bar Mitzvah is a very important rite of passage. It marks the transition from boyhood to manhood. At least ten men are required to hold a service and once a boy is Bar Mitzvah'd, he is counted as one of the ten men. But by 1972, when I came of age, Bar Mitzvahs had become so much less and so much more than that. Bar Mitzvahs no longer really signified passage into adulthood; after all, most boys have their Bar Mitzvah when they are in eighth grade. From my perspective, having attended several Bar Mitzvahs by then, the primary purpose was to give thirteen-year-old boys (and by then more and more often girls, too) a chance to shine in the spotlight by playing a major role in a Saturday service. And no less important, it gave parents a chance to bask in the glow of a child's accomplishment and then throw a really good party.

Had it been up to me, I wouldn't have had a Bar Mitzvah. The whole thing felt like a big act. And truly, it was. But not having one was never an option—mainly, it would have been a huge embarrassment to my parents. But also,

I didn't want to have to listen to the abuse I knew I would receive from my Hebrew School classmates if I chickened out.

The cantor of our synagogue was responsible for preparing me. When he was not singing, he was a quiet, kindly, older man. Aware of my reputation in Hebrew School, he was somewhat dubious about my willingness/ability to prepare properly. He became more doubtful about my commitment after I missed our first two sessions. At this point, my father stepped in and threatened to severely punish me if I didn't start taking Bar Mitzvah seriously. So I finally buckled down and got to work.

My Bar Mitzvah felt like a huge school project that culminated in me having to perform in front of a big room full of people. True, I would get lots of money and some nice gifts. But the work I needed to do to get ready for the event felt overwhelming. And I was terrified of having to perform in front of the entire congregation. I had to sing a twenty-minute passage from the Haftorah plus a five minute passage from the Torah, all in Hebrew. Having learned in Hebrew School how to read Hebrew text helped a little. But it didn't help that I had no idea what the words I was to sing meant. Preparing to sing these passages meant memorizing, syllable for syllable, a tape the cantor made of himself singing them. I must have played that tape a few hundred times before I felt I was ready.

Still, I had a major problem. One I could not overcome no matter how much I practiced. As Edye and Mandy frequently reminded me, I had an awful singing voice. I simply could not carry a tune. The only person we knew whose voice was worse than mine was my father. During regular services, I would just pretend to sing so no one would notice my voice. But during my Bar Mitzvah, mine would be the only voice in the congregation.

We arrived early on the day of my Bar Mitzvah and I tried to remain calm, but felt my heart beating way too fast. I sat in a chair on the altar behind the rabbi. The service began and I waited anxiously for what seemed like hours until, finally, my turn came. As I stepped to the lectern, I could feel my body shake. But once I started singing the Haftorah I became so focused that my anxiety melted away. Despite my terrible singing voice, I managed to give a credible performance. My parents were proud and I was relieved. But, with one notable exception, the whole exercise made me that much more cynical about religion.

A couple of weeks before my Bar Mitzvah I met with the synagogue's rabbi. I had been afraid of this man. He always seemed to have a scowl on his face and I was sure that every time I was a little slow to stand up or sit down during service he noticed me. I also was sure he knew I faked singing. I dreaded meeting with him. I expected the rabbi to start the meeting by dressing me down for not participating in the services. After that, I expected a lecture on the importance of my Bar Mitzvah: he would warn me that I was about to become a man, so I needed to pay better attention during services and start living a pious life.

But he surprised me. He greeted me with a warm smile and firm handshake. Then, he actually talked and listened to me in a way that acknowledged I had given some thought to what it meant to be a Jew. He answered my question about how the stories in the Bible could possibly be true by explaining that the stories were not meant to be taken literally. Some of the stories were parables and others were exaggerations that helped to simplify the telling of an actual event. The example that made the biggest impression on me was the story of how God parted the Red Sea so that the Israelites could escape from Pharaoh's soldiers. His explanation, that the Israelis passed through during a low tide and a calm sea, but the Pharaoh's men, arriving several hours later, faced a high tide and a stormy sea, seemed plausible to me. And for this to happen was no less a miracle than the literal story of the Red Sea parting.

This conversation had a profound impact on how I viewed religion. I no longer saw it as belief in a bunch of stories that could not possibly be true. I now understood that religious belief was far more subtle and complex and that perfectly reasonable, intelligent people could have strong religious beliefs. My skepticism remained about how each religion teaches its believers they are somehow different from and better than everyone else. But I now understood these teachings and the immoral acts they justified were something apart from the core belief in God as creator and moral overseer that all religions appear to share.

Still, at this point in my life I knew much more about what I didn't believe than what I did believe and I had a lot more questions than answers. It wasn't until college that I would start to develop my own set of beliefs.

· · · · · · · · ·

A Punch in the Gut

It hit me like a punch in the gut. Not that I was surprised. At thirteen, I was old enough to know something was up that morning when I saw my father had slept on a couch in the living room—something I had never seen him do before. Also, I had expected for some time that my parents would eventually split up. A few months earlier I had said out loud that they should get divorced. We were having dinner on a Sunday night at the Huki Lau restaurant, as we did every Sunday night. About halfway through the meal, no longer able to suppress my anger and embarrassment at my parents, I interrupted a loud argument by blurting out, "Why don't you just get divorced?" Suddenly, everyone at our table stopped talking, while the people at the next table uttered an audible gasp, as if they had just seen something scary in a horror movie. After a few very awkward moments my parents started talking again, but now in normal conversational voices. I immediately regretted making my comment, but nobody ever said anything to me about it. By the time we got home the tension had evaporated, as if I had never said anything. So that morning, several months later, when my father sat me down to "have a talk"—something he rarely did—I knew what he was about to tell me. Still, I wasn't prepared when my father spoke the words: "Your mother and I will not be living together anymore."

My father went on to say I should not blame my mother because he was mostly at fault. He then said my sisters and I would be living with our mother. As he talked, waves of numbness coursed through my body. My father continued to talk for a few more minutes, but I heard nothing else he said.

Dazed, I spent most of the next few days trying to make sense of it all. But I was unable to think it through logically, as I normally would when I experienced a set-back. Random thoughts about my mother, my father and what was going to happen to me raced through my head. I didn't know what to think.

During those first few days, I didn't reach out to any-one and no one reached out to me. It did not even occur to me to talk with either of my sisters and the last person in the world I wanted to talk to was my mother. I might have talked with my father, but he left for what I assumed to be another business trip soon after delivering the news.

Within a few days I reached the conclusion that it real-ly was all my mother's fault. Who could live with someone who always seemed to find something to yell about, and was so unattractive physically? I could hardly blame my father for wanting to get out; if anything, I wondered how he managed to stay as long as he did. I admired him for sitting me down, telling me about the break-up and tak-ing the blame, while my mother hadn't said a word to me about it.

Two or three days later, my mother announced we would be moving to Fairfield, Connecticut. The prospect of leaving Pittsfield, Massachusetts, did not upset me— with all the abuse I was taking from my peers, I had come to hate living there. But I was afraid of what my life would be like in Fairfield. I would be living with a mother I hated and who I thought hated me.

By then my sisters Edye and Mandy and I had acknowledged to each other that we had heard the news. It hung like a fog in our house, always present, impossible to ignore. I talked to my sisters, but never about how I felt, how I blamed my mother for everything, my fears about the future, or anything else that really mattered. And too wrapped up in my own thoughts, I didn't ask what they were thinking or how they were feeling. To all our detriment, we did not pull together and support each other. We lived in the same house, but in separate worlds. Each of us had to find his own way to deal with our parents' break-up.

The break-up must have been especially hard on Edye. As my father's favorite, she had a special relationship with him. Suddenly not having him around on a regular basis had to have been a huge loss to her. Fortunately, she had a couple of close friends with whom she could talk. But, two months shy of her twelfth birthday when she received the news, she also needed the support of an adult. Sadly, between my father's frequent extended absences and my mother's inability to see or feel anything beyond her own bitterness, no such adult existed to provide this support.

Mandy seemed to handle our parent's breakup better than Edye or me. Not having had a close relationship with our father for several years, his departure from our daily lives represented a smaller loss for her than for us. Also, fifteen at the time and accustomed to little or no parental supervision, Mandy had become very independent. But perhaps most important, Mandy had a wide circle of friends she could rely on for support.

I could not do that. Ashamed to admit my parents

had separated, I lied about it to my friends. I explained my father's absence by telling them he was away on business trips. It became almost like a game with John and his brother, David. The two of them told me they knew my parents had separated and I insisted they hadn't. They knew I was lying and I knew that they knew. Still, they persisted. I wanted them to stop. In retrospect I think they were just trying to help.

I continued to hide my parents' divorce until senior year of high school. When asked about my father, I would say he worked for General Electric. My questioners, aware that GE had its headquarters in Fairfield, assumed he worked there. I didn't bother to correct them. Mandy asked me once why I lied about my father. I couldn't answer her then and I still can't.

At first, I just wanted him back. That and how much blame my mother deserved were all I could think about. But after a few weeks, I began to see the larger picture. My father had walked out on not only my mother, but on my sisters and me as well. Despite being keenly aware of how little effort my mother put into being a parent and how bad my relationship with her had become, he gave no indication he had given even a moment's thought to having me live with him. I didn't dare ask because I knew the answer and I didn't want to experience the rejection of hearing it from him.

I started to resent my father and feel sorry for my mother. As a result, I abruptly changed my behavior towards her. I started going out of my way to be extra nice to her no matter what she said to me. Mandy and Edye, noticing the change, found it annoying and insincere. They told me to stop being such a phony. My mother didn't know what to make of it. But, grateful for any support, she accepted it. I frequently found myself gritting my teeth trying to be nice, but that made my behavior no less sincere. I really did feel sorry for my mother and I really did want to help.

During my mother's frequent tirades she occasionally shared a new concern: money. Here I saw an opportunity. I told my mother that if she got me a lawnmower, I would cut our lawn so she wouldn't have to pay the lawn service. I would then also have a lawnmower I could use to make some money for myself. I also asked my father. Incredulous at first, he pointed out that our lawn service and all of the neighbors on our side of the street used tractor mowers. Using a hand mower, our lawn would be a three to four hour job. But impressed with my entrepreneurship, he bought a lawnmower for me. True to my word, I cut our lawn every week.

Owning a lawnmower did enable me to make some money for myself, but not in the manner I expected. I started my job search by going up and down Tor Court, asking our neighbors if they needed someone to cut their lawns. Not a single one said yes. Undeterred, I extended my search to West Street, staying on the side of the street not facing the lake, with the more modest homes. After a few houses I hit pay dirt. An elderly woman opened her door and greeted me warmly. I started to make my pitch. But before I could finish she stopped me and said yes. She would like me to cut her lawn and she also would like me to help her with cleaning around her house, plus her lakefront cottage on Blythewood Drive. After intense negotiation, we agreed on four dollars for cutting her modestly-sized lawn and a dollar per hour for all other work. I knew she had driven a tough bargain—the minimum wage in 1972 was $1.60 an hour—but I was happy to have found regular work. She said she would like me to start right away so I ran home and came back with my lawnmower.

She gave me mostly easy work like dusting and vacuuming, often accompanying me to ensure that I did it correctly. But occasionally she gave me truly backbreaking work. One time, she asked me to clean out the chicken coop in her backyard. Another time she asked me to move a huge pile of dirt at her cottage. Both times I started the job, I realized how little she was paying me for the work I was doing, and demanded a raise to two dollars per hour. Fully aware she had been taking advantage of me, she relented and gave me the raise, at the same time reminding me it did not apply for indoor work. Although hardly a match made in heaven, our relationship worked out well for both of us.

Lony

Meanwhile, I began to wonder about the woman my father had left us for. My father hadn't so much as mentioned her existence. But my mother sure had. "She is a whore and a slut—a heartless bitch that ran out on her three young children," my mother repeated over and over again in her rants. My parents had not just "decided to live separately," as my father had told me when he gave me the news. He had said then that it was his fault and I didn't believe him, but now I knew he was right. He had left my mother for this woman. But who was this person who finally lured him away? As a fourteen-year-old with raging hormones I imagined her as a gorgeous temptress.

75

She'd better at least be good-looking, I thought.

I was alone with my father as he drove me to his rental house in Becket. He had boasted that the house was only a half hour away from his office and us. Plus, it was on a lake, so he could go sailing every evening after work. *Good for him*, I thought contemptuously. My father gave me no hint that Lony would be there. He opened the door and there she was, flitting about in the kitchen. I recoiled at the prospect of meeting her. But he and Lony had planned this non-introduction well. They both acted as if she and I had known each other forever. There was no need for an introduction. Lony and I didn't even acknowledge each other's presence.

I sat down in the living room while my father went to get something. *Great*, I thought. Now I can check her out. I watched her closely, making sure she didn't catch my eye as I waited for my father to return. Lony certainly was attractive, but she looked nothing like the whore of my mother's tirades or the temptress of my fantasies. She was wore a loose-fitting T-shirt and patterned knee-length shorts. She had a pretty but not striking face framed by straight blond hair that curled inward a couple of inches above her shoulders. She was shapely, but not like the Playboy models whose pictures I had stashed in my room. She appeared to be perhaps five to ten years younger than my father—not a big enough difference to make people notice. As she moved about the kitchen, putting away dishes and preparing a meal, she reminded me a little of Doris Day. All in all, I thought she was an attractive, respectable-looking woman.

When my father returned a few minutes later, Lony

announced in a pleasant but heavily-accented voice that lunch was ready. I couldn't make out the accent then, but later learned it was Dutch. The three of us sat down at the table, me with my head down to avoid making eye contact. Lony's body language was open and friendly. Mine screamed that I wanted to be someplace else. When Lony asked me what I wanted to drink or whether I wanted more to eat, I responded with one-word answers.

Mandy's introduction to Lony must have been even more awkward than mine. My parents threw a number of parties with upwards of a hundred guests at our house on Tor Court. Our huge downstairs family room, with its full kitchen and sliders leading out to the back yard, made our house the perfect venue for a party of this size. My mother, proud of her cooking skills, basked in the praise she received for catering these parties herself. One party I remember well took place on New Year's Eve 1970. Many of my parents' guests were more than a little tipsy by the time the clock struck midnight. I saw several of my parents' friends in a whole new light that night.

But the most raucous parties were the ones my parents threw for my father's work colleagues. At one party several guests, drunk, went down to the lake and jumped in, fully clothed. Another one of these parties took place shortly before my parents separated. During this party, Mandy noticed my father spending most of his time with an attractive blond. The way my father and this woman looked at and touched each other signified a relationship that went far beyond casual flirting. This attractive blond was, of course, Lony. Mandy knew who Lony was even before they met.

Thankfully, I did not learn of this incident until long after my father died. It bothered me, but not nearly as much as it would have had I witnessed it. Still, I am amazed at my father's—and Lony's—audacity. Mandy clearly was not the only person who noticed the two of them. Everyone at the party would also have noticed. Also, Pittsfield being a small, insular community, anyone in my parents' social circle not at that party would have found out soon enough. My mother, of course, also had to have known what was going on. Worse than that, she had to have known that everyone else in her social circle knew as well. She must have felt thoroughly humiliated. It is easy to see why she became so bitter.

Mandy's introduction to Lony must have gone off without fireworks because I never heard anything about it. I just knew that within a few weeks of my meeting Lony, both Mandy and Edye had met her as well.

Near the end of summer my father told me he had taken a new position with General Electric in Milwaukee. But before I could get too upset, he also told me he had bought a nearby cottage on Onota Lake. He explained he planned to winterize and expand the cottage so it would be a comfortable place for us to visit any time of year.

Moving with My Mother

My mother wanted to move back to Fairfield, Connecticut, where we had lived for several years in the early 1960s. Her plan was to move before the start of the school year, but before she could buy a new house there, she had to sell our house on Tor Court. Unfortunately, not many buyers existed in Pittsfield who could afford a house like ours, so it did not sell quickly. My sisters and I began the school year in Pittsfield.

School began and I returned a changed person. I no longer made inappropriate comments, refused to do my work, or played the role of class clown. No longer wanting to be the center of attention, I became the quietest kid in class. I just wanted to be left alone. A few of my class-mates, surprised by my new persona, asked me why I had changed. But I couldn't bring myself to tell them about my parents' divorce, so I just made up a story.

Still in Pittsfield when the Jewish High Holy Days arrived, my mother, sisters, and I went to synagogue for Yom Kippur services. We had been sitting through the service for perhaps an hour when I saw my father arrive. He saw us and sat down near us, making me very uncomfortable. I then became an unwilling actor in a drama that I remember almost as a dream. I was seated with my mother on my left and my sisters on my right. A couple I didn't know occupied the two seats to the right of my sisters. My father sat down in an empty seat next to this couple. After a few minutes, both Edye and Mandy got up to take a break. My father then moved over and sat next to me, so now I had my mother on one side and my father on the other. Then, in a show of solidarity, Mother put her hand on my left hand. A few moments later, my father took hold of my right hand.

To someone who didn't know them well, this gesture might be interpreted as an act of love by my parents, each holding a hand to reassure me that, even though they didn't love each other anymore, they still shared their love for me. But this interpretation could not be further from the truth. In reality, it was a childish, petty act, mostly on the part of my father, but also by my mother, to show the congregation that (s)he was the parent that had a special bond with his/her child. This incident would be the first of countless more in which one of my sisters or I would suffer the collateral damage caused by my parents' unending post-marriage battles.

In a final act of anger and petulance, I didn't tell anyone at school I was leaving until my final day. Even then I told only one person, Joe, who had become my best friend at school. The football team played its first game that day. I suited up like everyone else and boarded the bus to the game against our cross-town rival. Our team won a close, emotional game, while I sat on the bench. On the entire ride home I sat in silence, alone in my thoughts, unlike my cheering teammates. Upon arriving back at Crosby, I quickly changed out of my uniform and got dressed. I then gave one of the assistant coaches my uniform and pads, telling him I was quitting the team. Then I left without saying so much as goodbye to the few friends I had on the team. We moved to Fairfield the next day.

CHAPTER 6
MOVE TO FAIRFIELD

For most of my adult life, I remembered my second stay in Fairfield as a four-year nightmare. My mother's behavior toward me sunk to a new low that bordered on criminal, I had no friends, and my classmates abused me almost non-stop—mostly verbally, but sometimes physically. When I thought about this time—something I did often—I never remembered anything good about it. How I managed to emerge from college only four years later self-assured, well-liked and respected by my peers, and having an academic record that promised a bright future had been a mystery to me. But sometimes our memories can play tricks on us. Yes, most of the people I regularly saw and interacted with didn't treat me very well. And that made it a difficult, often very painful time for me. But I also met a few people who accepted, respected and even loved me. I also experienced some moments of unexpected kindness and caring from some of the people who treated me most harshly. It gives me comfort now to know that even during this awful time of my life, I persisted and found moments of joy and happiness.

I also now realize that high school was a time of enormous personal growth for me. I gained a sense of self-identity. I gained the courage to stand up for myself when necessary. I gained confidence in my resiliency. And I learned to appreciate small kindnesses. I didn't magically turn my life around during college. I started in small ways even before moving to Fairfield. And by the time I got to college, I was already well on my way.

Our Transition to Fairfield

Our new house, a modestly sized four-bedroom, center-hall colonial with a postage-stamp-sized yard, was a world apart from 73 Tor Court. Located only about a half mile from the edge of Bridgeport—a city that had long since begun its decline and which Paul Newman had called "the armpit of New England"—our house was part of a solidly middle-class, residential neighborhood. While not at all a bad place to live, it was at the low end of the scale for Fairfield.

My room, a finished porch, was just large enough to fit my bed and a small table, which housed the stereo I bought with the money I earned the previous summer. While lying in bed, I could almost reach the opposite wall. Drawers built into my bed served as a dresser.

At first I liked my new home. I preferred its coziness to the isolation I often felt at 73 Tor Court. I also liked no longer being in the spotlight. I even preferred the blue collar feel of the neighborhood.

Shortly after moving into the house I discovered a park a few blocks away. A basketball court in the park attracted a cast of characters from a wide area, stretching from my neighborhood well into Bridgeport. This park was not a place for rich kids and I preferred it that way. Our pick-up games were often intense, with lots of hard fouls and arguing, but I cannot recall a single fight breaking out.

I felt an unspoken bond with these guys, a sense of mutual recognition that nothing came easy to any of us. Whether anyone else felt this bond, I will never know.

. . . .

My mother, sisters, and I spent the first two days in Fairfield unpacking, happily delaying the start of school. I would start as a freshman. My self-confidence was at an all-time low. I dreaded starting out all over again. I wished we could put off school for just a few more days, and after that, perhaps another week.

Early the next morning, my wishes having gone unanswered, I headed off with Mandy to Andrew Warde High School. Fifteen minutes into our walk, the building came into view. It seemed to stretch on forever. Shaped like an airport terminal, the building had four wings connected by a main hallway. We passed two of these wings on our way to the main entrance.

By the time we got into the building I could feel sweat trickling down from my armpits and my steps becoming unsteady. Mandy seemed unfazed, as if she had done this several times before. "Where do we go now?" I asked her. "How will I find my classes? What courses do I take? Does anybody from the school even know we are supposed to be here?"

Making no attempt to hide her annoyance, Mandy replied, "Stop worrying so much." I secretly wanted her to hold my hand. Mandy found the main office, walked in while I followed closely behind, and told the receptionist our names. Evidently expecting us, she welcomed us and then quickly completed a form she had sitting on her desk. Next she explained the high school was divided into three "houses." I was to report to the Walcott House office and Mandy to the Barlow House office. The receptionist gave us directions and sent us on our way. I begged Mandy to take me to the Walcott House office and she reluctantly complied. There, I met with a guidance counselor who gave me more information about the school and handed me my class schedule. The rest of the day was a blur.

My parents' divorce had transformed me from someone who reveled in the attention of being the class clown to a frightened ninth grader who just wanted to be left alone. I had become shy and socially awkward, retreating so far into myself that meeting anyone new had become a painful experience.

. . . .

My social discomfort caused me to miss a golden opportunity to reconnect with an old friend. During the first few weeks of school, preferring not sitting over sitting next to someone I didn't know, I spent the entire twenty-five-minute lunch period walking back and forth from one end of the cafeteria to the other. One day, perhaps a week or two after starting at Andrew Warde, a very attractive girl came up to me during my daily amble through the cafeteria. She smiled at me and said, "Ira, do you remember me? I'm Cheryl. We knew each other when we were little kids."

Of course I remembered her. My first true love, Cheri, lived on our side of the street two or three houses away.

Cheri, a small, athletic girl, had sandy brown hair she wore up in curls. Even through the lenses of my six-year-old eyes I could tell she was quite pretty. That wasn't all that attracted me to her, though. I also liked that she was not the prissy type—Cheri liked to climb trees, ride bikes, and do other little boy activities.

One day at Cheri's house I offered her some M&Ms I had brought from my house. Cheri's mother gave me a warm smile and told me I was a generous person. Confused, I thanked her anyway. My parents—mainly my mother—called me names all the time. But never with a smile. I knew what "moron" and "stupid" and "idiot" meant but I had never before heard the word generous. When I found out its meaning I walked around with my chest puffed out for the next several days.

Cheri and I planned to get married, and not just for play. We meant it. For an engagement ring I gave her a paper ring from one of my father's cigars. She happily accepted it. However, Cheri's mother, who strongly supported the marriage, suggested we wait until we became grown-ups for the big day. Cheri and I reluctantly agreed. But within the next year my father announced we were moving to a bigger house in another part of town. Cheri and I said a tearful goodbye, never expecting to see each other again. I lost track of her when my family moved away from Barry Scott Drive, but I could never forget her.

And now here she was, a beautiful girl welcoming me to reminisce with her. But all I could manage was "Oh yeah. I remember you," as my feet shuffled back and forth, advertising my discomfort.

Cheryl responded in a friendly voice, "Well, it's so nice to see you again," giving me a second chance to keep the conversation going.

I wanted to tell her how wonderful a surprise it was to see her again. I wanted to share a laugh with her over our childhood marriage plans. I wanted to get to know her again and possibly become friends. But I just said, "Yeah, it's been great to see you again," while telling her with my body language that I desperately wanted the conversation to end.

After an awkward moment she said, "See ya around," and walked away. I saw her a few more times and once almost gathered the courage to go up to her and try to start a conversation, but we never spoke to each other again.

. . . .

During the entire four years I had lived in Pittsfield, even with all the abuse boys heaped on me, not a single girl ever teased or otherwise put me down. It was almost as if they were unaware of my lowly status among the boys. I got along well with girls in my classes and usually found it easy to talk with them.

My experience at Andrew Warde could not have been more different. Within a matter of days a couple of girls in my French class, Lisa and Peggy, started teasing me. They mockingly told me—and the rest of the class—that they wanted to have sex with me. "Any time," they would say, "I'm ready whenever you are." If one of them caught me looking at her, she would wink or blow a kiss at me. I said "Fuck you" to Lisa once and she replied, "Okay."

I can now see why Lisa and Peggy picked on me. If it is true that people can smell fear, then I reeked of it. I sat low in my chair, not speaking unless spoken to. Whenever my eyes met with someone, I quickly looked down. I fidgeted constantly.

I might have gone unnoticed had it not been for my French teacher, Mr. V. He would go around the class in no particular order, asking and expecting people to answer questions in French. He subjected anyone who couldn't answer to an interrogation until he or she replied to his satisfaction. Despite having taken French in Pittsfield, my understanding of the language was well below expectations for this class. I couldn't answer Mr. V. He relentlessly rode me, chiding me for my inability to respond to even the easiest questions. One time he even asked me if everyone from Pittsfield was stupid.

With a considerable amount of studying, I finally got out of Mr. V's cross-hairs. But Lisa's and Peggy's teasing continued unabated. I racked my brain trying to find a way to get them to stop until one day I had an answer. As we sat waiting for Mr. V to start class, Peggy said "Oh baby, I want you."

I replied, with the whole class listening, "The problem with you and Lisa is that you're all talk and no action." The class broke into laughter. Even Mr. V laughed. I had called their bluff. They tried teasing me a few times afterwards, but each time I answered similarly. "You keep telling me that," I might say. "When do you want to get together?" Within a few days, they stopped.

I can attribute my difficulties in Mr. V's class at least partly to bad luck. But I have only myself to blame for the reputation I made for myself in geometry class. A couple of days after starting school, I learned Andrew Warde offered a fast track for the smartest kids in math and science. The kids in this track took courses a year ahead of the rest of their class. In addition, they took more advanced versions of these courses. A freshman, I found myself in a geometry class with sophomores. This meant that, although I was taking the same course as the fast-track kids, I was not in the fast track.

That bugged me. I still considered myself to be a star in math—in fact, my math skills were the main source of what little self-confidence I had at the time. The next day I asked my guidance counselor if I could switch to the advanced class. Visibly annoyed, she reminded me I had just started this class a month into the semester and I had plenty of catching up to do. I persisted and she repeated she did not want me to switch, this time letting me know by the tone in her voice that the conversation was over.

Since repeating kindergarten, I needed to prove I could "play with the big boys." By not allowing me to take the advanced math class, my guidance counselor had denied me this opportunity. So I set out to show her, my teacher, and the rest of the class that I belonged in the advanced class, that I was too smart to be in a class with students who were just average. Whenever my teacher asked a question, I made sure to raise my hand before anyone else. I let everyone know I didn't need to do the homework assignments because I could solve problems on the fly. I frequently commented that the class was too easy. Blinded by my need to prove I belonged in the advanced class, I never considered how my classmates might perceive this behavior. In the process, I established myself as being the only thing worse than a nerd: an arrogant nerd.

Meanwhile, at home, we picked up where we had left off in Pittsfield, my mother resuming her frequent outbursts and Edythe, Mandy, and me each retreating to our own separate worlds. My mother added self-pity to her repertoire and began yelling at no one in particular. "After seventeen years," she would wail, "this is the thanks I get from him?" Or, "Now I'm a fifth wheel; no one will invite me to go anywhere with them." Or—my personal favorite—"I could have moved in to a three-room apartment, but instead I'm stuck with, with"—now waving her arms toward one of my sisters or me—"this."

For the first time, she included concerns about money in her rants. "I can't stand it," she would cry. "Everything is so expensive. How am I supposed to make ends meet?" She had a good point—it did cost more to live in Fairfield than in Pittsfield. She received just enough from the sale of our huge lakefront house in Pittsfield to make a down payment on our modest home in Fairfield and leave a small cushion for unanticipated expenses. And with her shopping habits, her monthly alimony and child support payments really were just enough to get by.

My mother spent a sizable chunk of her nest egg on dental care for me. She took me to our dentist—a close friend of my parents the first time we lived in Fairfield—for a routine check-up. He told us I had twenty-one cavities, which would require several visits to fill. It didn't cross my mind that this dental work could be expensive and my mother never told me how much it cost. But shortly after my check-up she began including in her rants, "That bastard. And I thought he was my friend. Friends are supposed to help each other out."

At first, I tried to empathize with my mother or at least not pay attention to her tirades. I also continued to look for ways to help out. But her near-constant harping about how badly my father had mistreated her, made worse by a screeching voice that at times sounded like crows squawking after discovering an open bag of garbage, became impossible for me to ignore. At least my father, for all his faults, never said anything bad about my mother. The anger I felt towards her began to boil to the surface. Finally, after one too many tirades about my father, followed by "and you, you, you're just like him," I cracked. I couldn't remain silent anymore. I started yelling back at her.

I yelled at my mother to "just shut up and leave me alone," hoping without reason that she would relent and stop her harangues just long enough to give me a little peace and quiet. But, of course, my yelling back had exactly the opposite effect. My mother stepped up her attacks on me. And I yelled louder at her to stop, as if raising my voice would make a difference. It took no more than a day or two for our relationship to regress to where it had been before I started to sympathize with her. We no longer talked to each other in a normal conversational voice. Yelling at each other had become our sole means of communication. We had begun to explore the depths to which our relationship would go.

CHAPTER 7
LIVING TO RUN AND RUNNING TO LIVE

Many teenagers have a special place where they can go to be by themselves and try to make sense of the world. I didn't go to a special place when I needed to be by myself; I went running.

I started running during the summer before ninth grade to get in shape for football. I knew we would be moving from Pittsfield soon. But I had always liked—and been pretty good at—pick-up football, so I decided to go out for the Andrew Warde team. We spent the first week of practice just doing exercises to get in shape. Like everyone else, I hated the wind sprints. But I enjoyed the one mile run we did at the beginning and end of each practice. In excellent shape from my summer running, I found myself at the front of the pack. I was a star! But then, in the second week, our coaches started us on the hitting drills. I soon realized I didn't like hitting all that much and I hated getting hit. The coaches noticed my aversion to hitting, and so found a nice safe place for me at the end of the bench.

Still under the illusion I had some athletic talent, I tried out for the freshman basketball and baseball teams at Andrew Warde. I was a first-round cut in both sports. Next, having forgotten my lesson from the previous fall, I went out for spring football. Big mistake! I had no more affinity for hitting and getting hit then than I had six months earlier. This time my misadventure with football turned out to be a truly humiliating experience. We all started the workouts wearing plain white jerseys, and as each player made the team, he received a crimson-red—the school color—jersey. Between the freshman, sophomore, and junior classes about seventy-five kids participated in the spring practices. I was one of only three that didn't earn a crimson jersey.

I loved sports. I knew I had to do something. After giving it some thought, I realized that the only part of football I actually liked was the running. So I decided to give running a try. I started running every evening after dinner, first just around the neighborhood for maybe a mile and, by the middle of summer, up to three miles at a time. The more I ran the easier it became and the more I liked it. I resolved to run cross country in the fall. I knew I would make the team because no one got cut from cross country. And this time, being in shape from my summer running would actually make a difference. To my surprise, I discovered I was actually pretty decent. We had a terrible team, so it didn't take much to be pretty decent, but still, I was one of the better runners on the team. I had finally found my niche as an athlete.

It is hard to overstate just how bad our team was. Made up of non-conformists, misfits, and people like me who just wanted to participate in a sport, any sport, our team had maybe twenty-five runners, only four or five of whom could accurately be described as athletes. The team's coach, Mr. C, was missing in action most of the time and when he did show up he would ramble incoherently for several minutes and then tell us to get out there and run. We were completely directionless.

Then one day a guy showed up who looked like a hippie in shorts and track shoes. He had long blond hair and a full beard. Clearly too old to be a student, he also didn't look like any teacher I knew. I later found out he taught in the Outward Bound program. Unlike every other teacher, he asked us to use his first name, introducing himself as John. He told us he would be leading our runs. John turned out to be exactly the guy he appeared to be at first glance—a running hippie. He also turned out to be one of those people who made a big difference in my life just when I needed it most.

Steeped in Eastern thought, John made it an essential component of his coaching philosophy. He spoke of the yin and yang and the importance of keeping these opposing forces in balance. He taught us to just have fun and not to worry about how fast or slow we ran. He told us it didn't matter whether we won or lost the race as long as we enjoyed the journey. He had a willing group of disciples. Most of us had gained some familiarity with Eastern thought by watching the hit TV show *Kung Fu* and were ready to learn more. Also, many on the team were overjoyed to hear they didn't have to run hard. We loved our new running guru.

Rather than have us do structured workouts like every other team, John led us in a series of fun runs. He called one of these runs the Comet Vomit: we ran to the Comet Diner, about two and a half miles away, ate an ice cream sundae, and ran back. He called another the Popsicle Run. For this run, we stopped at a convenience store about a mile and a half before the end of the run, bought a popsicle and tried to finish the run before the popsicle melted.

I never quite understood the point of yin and yang but I loved running. It felt good to be able to run at an easy pace for several miles without even feeling tired. I also liked the kind of tired I felt after pushing myself on a hard run. But for me it wasn't entirely about the journey. Despite John's advice, I took the races very seriously.

In cross-country, each school has its own course. Before each away meet, we went over as much of the course as we could by bus and jogged the rest. Most of the guys on the team goofed off as we went over the course but I paid rapt attention, carefully plotting my strategy. My team mates often made fun of me for my intensity. I didn't like that they picked on me but their jibes just made me more intense.

When the season ended, John offered to continue to meet after school with anyone interested in going on some longer runs. Only three of us took him up on the offer. Joining me were Greg, the only guy on our team who could compete with the better runners in the conference, and his older brother Bill, the second fastest runner on our team. The four of us ran together every day. We gradually increased our distance until finally we completed an eighteen-mile run. We didn't just jog on these runs. We ran hard. We started out slowly and after two or three miles, John and Greg would gradually increase the pace until Bill and I could no longer keep up. Trying not to finish too much later than John and Greg, Bill and I would continue to run at a solid but manageable pace the rest of the way.

Each time we ran a little further I felt a little more confident, and not just about running. I didn't realize it at the time, but these runs changed my life. I no longer ran to get in shape or even to prepare for a race. Running had become an important part of my self-identity. Finally, I had something other than math to feel good about. I gained not only confidence, but also a feeling of strength from being a runner. How many other people could run— not just jog, really run—eighteen miles? I felt almost invincible, that I could accomplish anything I set my mind to. This confidence, bordering on arrogance, stayed with me for the next thirty years.

We stopped these runs a few weeks before the start of indoor track season. By now, needing my daily fix of running, I couldn't wait for track to start. I started running again every night after dinner. I ran every day no matter how I felt. My only concession, if I felt really awful, was to shorten my run.

When indoor track finally started, I signed up for the mile and the two-mile run. By then I saw running as my niche, and not only in sports. As the Bob Seger song goes, I was living to run and running to live. I had forgotten about the yin and the yang and the rest of John's teachings and became very serious about track. Way too serious. I started to equate my success on the track with my success as a person. How I performed as a runner became far more important to me than how I performed academically.

Realizing I wasn't the most talented guy on the team, I made it my mission to work harder than anyone else. I thought that if I worked hard enough I might some-day become good enough to run in the Olympics. In fact, I counted on that because I didn't see any other path to success.

Our track coach paid scant attention to the distance

runners, making us as directionless as the cross country team had been under Mr. C. So when an opportunity came up to do real workouts, I jumped at it. Tom, a senior on our team, had won the state title in the quarter mile run the previous year. Like everyone else I revered him for his accomplishment. But I wondered how he could do so well because he never seemed to run very hard in practice. Then I learned that he did his serious workouts under his father's tutelage at Fairfield's other high school. He and his father invited a few of the better runners on our team to join him. Normally, someone at the top of the social pecking order would not even deign to speak to someone with my lowly status. But I mustered up the courage to ask Tom if I could join them and Tom, who I later learned had a measure of respect for me for my willingness to push myself, said yes. I didn't mind always being behind every-one during these workouts because I felt honored to have been accepted into this elite group and I loved the feeling of pushing myself to the limit.

Even while doing these workouts, I continued to do my evening runs. I did so not because I thought the extra running would make me more successful, but because I enjoyed the time I spent by myself running. It had become a kind of therapy. While running, I thought through whatever problems were bothering me at the time. When especially upset about something I would run as hard as I could so that by the time I finished, exhausted, I had released most of my anger and frustration.

Despite all my hard work, I never did become a track star. Unfortunately, both speed and stamina are required to be competitive in the mile and two-mile runs. I lacked speed. My best times in high school were 5:08 in the mile and 11:04 in the two-mile. To put these times in perspective, the better runners in my school's conference ran between 4:25 and 4:30 in the mile and under 9:50 in the two-mile. By my senior year I realized the only way I would get to the Olympics would be to buy a ticket.

As my dreams of glory on the track faded, I started thinking about one day running a marathon. The running boom hadn't started yet and running a marathon was not as commonplace as it is today. The Boston Marathon had fewer than 2,500 runners in 1976, the spring of my senior year, not the tens of thousands it has today. I thought that just completing a marathon, regardless of my time, would be a huge accomplishment. I made that goal the first thing on my list of things to do within my lifetime.

CHAPTER 8
THE FIGHT(S)

Between the Parents

By the end of our first year in Fairfield, money had become one of the main topics of conversation for the Fried family. We discussed this topic as we did most topics: by screaming at each other. My mother yelled at me daily for "eating like a pig." I heard her wail "I could have lived in a three-room apartment" so often that it almost became a mantra. She snapped at Edythe every time she mentioned she needed new clothes.

My mother was scared, and for good reason. She'd never had to manage a household on a tight budget before. And to make matters worse, I really did eat like a pig. My mother always served a substantial dinner, which I topped off with Twinkies, Cupcakes, or some other Hostess delicacy. On a typical day, I complemented dinner with two or three large bowls of cereal, a couple of pieces of fruit, and copious amounts of peanut butter, which I ate with a spoon directly from the industrial-sized, economy plastic tub my mother bought.

Learning to manage a budget with a teen-age boy/eating machine in the house was but a part of the challenge my mother faced. From the shards of information I picked up from listening to my parents argue, I believe my mother's divorce attorney to have been at best incompetent and possibly worse. By contrast, my father, himself very experienced at negotiating financial arrangements, hired an attorney he knew to be highly competent from collaborations with him on complex deals at work. It was an unfair fight. And my father pressed his advantage at every opportunity.

Negotiations over the divorce settlement dragged on for months after we moved. My mother's small nest egg gradually shrank as she paid her lawyer's fees. My mother lost on every important point, some with devastating consequences. For example, her child support payments stayed fixed at $35 per child per week for the entire time we lived in Fairfield, despite the fact that inflation began a steep climb at about the same time my parents were finalizing the divorce settlement. No wonder my mother's worry about money grew more intense each year.

My father continued to take advantage, even after signing the divorce settlement. His decision to cut off child support payments for Mandy and me during the summers we lived with him was the most egregious, but not the only example. He had to have understood that my mother had expenses, like mortgage and utility payments, that didn't go away when one of us lived with him temporarily. My mother, no longer able to afford an attorney, was powerless to do anything about it.

It is easy to see now how difficult my father made it for my mother. But as a fifteen-year-old, I had no appreciation of the fear gripping my mother, so I had little empathy for her. When she yelled at me that I was "eating her out of house and home," I just yelled back and kept on eating.

Years later, Lony told me my father's side of the story. She said my father wanted my mother to become independent. He reasoned that my mother had many talents and if she wanted to, could have gone back to school and started a career. Lony added that my father even offered to pay for her tuition. But my mother never took him up on his offer. She preferred to whine about how badly she had been mistreated and how miserable her life had become.

I can understand my father's reasoning. My mother did have many gifts. She had the organizational skills to cater parties with a hundred or more guests. Having acted in numerous plays, often in the lead role, she could speak comfortably in front of large groups of people. She had demonstrated strong leadership skills as the former president of her B'nai B'rith chapter. With some additional formal schooling to round out her resume, she could have been highly marketable.

However, my father's plans for my mother, in addition to being self-serving, failed to take into account her emotional state. She had shown remarkable resiliency each time they moved to advance my father's career. But, her confidence now drained, she was simply incapable of taking on a project as large as starting a career.

My father also failed to take into account the impact using money as a weapon had on my mother, my sisters, and me. After their arguments, my mother would invariably become hysterical, lashing out at anyone in her path. Mandy and Edythe usually managed to avoid the worst of my mother's wrath, but I always seemed to walk right into it. My mother and I both needed an outlet for our anger and self-loathing and we chose each other.

Between Me and Mike

During the fall of sophomore year, I began to notice a major shift taking place at school. The countercultural ethos, which had been on its last legs during freshman year, gradually but inexorably faded and jock culture reasserted its dominance. This change was most apparent in the way people dressed. During freshman year, guys who wanted to look cool donned ratty-looking clothes, like faded jeans with patches and tears, old army jackets, and worn-out work boots. They wore their hair long and, if they could, grew lots of facial hair. By the middle of my sophomore year, all but a small contingent of pot-heads and rebels had cut their hair and gotten rid of their beards and mustaches. Crisp new blue jeans and painters' pants replaced torn, faded jeans. Rugby shirts became all the rage.

The accompanying change in attitude, although less noticeable at first, had a much greater impact on me. People rarely talked about religious beliefs or causes—like peace and civil rights—that recently had seemed so important. Popularity in the jock culture required maintaining an air of cool indifference. An attitude of apathy prevailed. If we'd had a school motto it would have been "Who cares?" The jock culture demanded conformity. Those who didn't conform, whether intentionally or not, became outcasts.

I stood out like a sore thumb. I wore out-of-style, ill-fitting clothes. My hair, way too long and festooned with cowlicks, looked matted and disheveled. But worst of all, I cared. I cared about getting into the advanced math courses. I cared about how well I did in cross country and track. I cared about religion and whether God existed. My attitude, social awkwardness, and appearance made me a prime target for bullies. It seemed that wherever I went people made fun of me, and worse. But having gained confidence from running I was now better prepared to handle bullying than ever before.

The taunting was especially brutal in English class. Mike, a football player wannabe with a pimpled face and enough grease in his long black hair to cook a batch of French fries, led the charge. Whenever the teacher was not paying attention, which was most of the time, Mike would hurl insults at me. Several others in the class would goad Mike on and occasionally throw some insults of their own my way.

Finally, the situation reached a boiling point. Our teacher left the room for a few minutes and Mike stepped up his attack, with several others gleefully joining in and the rest of the class watching. I lost my temper and threw an eraser at Mike, missing his head by a couple of inches. Before Mike could respond our teacher returned.

By the end of class, Mike had issued a challenge to fight. I dreaded the prospect, but knew I had no choice. I had run away from too many fights. Had I backed down from this one, I would have lost whatever shred of self-respect I had left. Mike and I agreed to the next day after school by the baseball field as the time and place.

That gave me an entire day to worry and plenty of time for word of the fight to get around school. I left English class that day with a lump in my throat that stayed with me until school ended the next afternoon. Not having a friend I could talk to or an adult I could trust, I was utterly alone in my fear.

When school ended the next day, I went to the locker
room to change into shorts and a T-shirt. Then I headed—
alone—to the baseball field. When I got to within fifty
yards I saw a crowd of thirty to forty jocks, heads, and low-
lifes straggling along the first base line. They saw me too
and started yelling that Mike was going to "kick my ass"
and "fuck me over real bad." I walked the rest of the way,
trying to stop my body from shaking, while praying that a
teacher would see the commotion and stop the fight. But
I would not be rescued this time. The catcalls grew louder
as I approached home plate, where Mike stood waiting for
me. Among the jeering and insults, I heard a few in the
crowd chanting, "Kill the Jew. Kill the Jew." I knew one of
them to be Jewish.

Mike and I both weighed about 140 pounds, but while
Mike stored his into a 5'6" bundle of muscle, I stretched
my weight over a 5'10" string bean frame. Everyone there,
including me, expected Mike to kick the crap out of me. I
wanted so badly to turn around and run back to the building, but knew I couldn't. Finally, Mike and I stood facing
each other. He spit in my face and the fight began.

I tried to move around and throw jabs, as if I were
Muhammad Ali. I managed to connect a few times but,
to my horror, saw that all of my punches were slaps. The
crowd laughed at me and urged Mike on. My strategy of
floating like a butterfly and stinging like a ... bee was not
working. Knowing I would get killed if I tried to box toe-
to-toe with Mike, I bull-rushed him and wrestled him to
the ground.

We have all heard stories of how, in emergencies, people have demonstrated superhuman strength, like lifting

up the end of a car to let out someone trapped underneath. What happened to me wasn't quite as dramatic as that but the adrenaline of the moment did seem to make me stronger than usual.

For what seemed like an hour, but must have been closer to fifteen minutes, I stayed on top of Mike, where he could not hurt me. The crowd yelled at Mike to get up and at me to fight the right way. After a few minutes on top of Mike, the shouts and screams had blurred into a cacophony of hate. But several times I heard one or two distinct voices shout at me that I was choking Mike and I could kill him if I didn't let up. I complied each time, releasing Mike from my choke-hold and quickly putting him in another hold before he could escape.

There were several close calls. One time he made it to his feet, but before he could ready himself, I pulled his feet out from under him, causing him to fall on his back. I then pounced on him, retaking my position on top. I had countless opportunities to punch or elbow him in the face, with the leverage to cause serious injury. But I couldn't do it.

I just wanted the fight to end. I asked Mike in a voice several decibels below the din of the crowd if he would leave me alone if I let him up. He answered succinctly: "Fuck you!" I pushed his face into the dirt and asked again. He replied, "I'm going to kill you when I get up." I pushed his face into the dirt again—this time hard enough to hurt—and beseeched him, "C'mon, Mike. I don't want to hurt you. We have nothing left to prove. I'm going to let you up and you're going to leave me alone. Okay?"

Just as I was about to push Mike's face into the dirt

again he grunted his approval to my offer. I got up to one knee and then released Mike as I stood up. I started to walk away, but before my second step Mike stood in front of me and punched me in the face, hard. I kept walking, offering no defense. It took everything I had to not break into a run. After landing two or three more solid punches Mike stopped. I continued walking until I got to the gym.

Feeling as if my conscious self had become detached from my body, I wandered to the room where the cross country team prepared for its daily run. I thought I would run with the team, as I did every day. Not until I tried to do a push-up did I realize how much the fight had taken out of me—I could not do even one.

I heard someone say in a sympathetic tone, "Go home, Ira." I did so, and as I walked the mile and a quarter to my house I contemplated what had happened. Why did I not try to hurt Mike when I had the chance? Why did Mike let me go after he landed his three or four punches? Who would people say won the fight?

The next day in English class Mike said very little to me, and with him no longer leading the charge, I didn't get the normal abuse. After school I went to the locker room to get changed for cross country practice. As usual right after school, the locker room was filled with people changing out of their school clothes and into their workout attire. Everybody there had to have either watched or heard about the fight. A couple of people said something complimentary to me, but I didn't hear a word about the fight from anyone else. From that I surmised most of them thought I had won.

Mike and I settled into an uneasy truce. I never asked

him why he stopped hitting me. My guess is that, humiliated from my holding him down until I decided to let him get up, he felt even more shame when I just walked away as he hit me. So he stopped.

I still sometimes wonder about the answer to my first question: Why did I not try to hurt Mike? Am I by nature a non-violent person, incapable of hurting another human being? Decades later, I told this story to some friends in a writing class. One of them said my actions demonstrated a spiritual nature. Another said my behavior was Gandhi-like. Perhaps. But I doubt that Gandhi would have replayed the fight over and over again in his mind, imagining he had fought back and seriously injured Mike, as I did for years afterwards.

The fight was a major milestone for me. I had finally stood up to a bully and won. I wish I could say the fight turned my life around, but unfortunately life is not always so simple. I gained a modicum of respect by winning the fight. And perhaps, as a result, I avoided being harassed by a succession of bullies. But I did not gain acceptance. The verbal abuse continued and only grew worse over my remaining two and a half years in high school.

CHAPTER 9
A COUPLE POINTS OF LIGHT IN HELL

My So-Called Friends

My social life improved slightly during junior year, as I became part of a small group of friends from the cross country team. The guys in this group—Lou, Jack, Greg and Phil, plus occasionally a few others—included me much of the time they got together. I regularly sat with them at lunch. Also, all of us avid basketball players, we frequently got together to play pick-up games on weekday evenings in the winter when schools held open gyms. And we played together on a rec league team in my junior and senior years.

But they also made me feel like a pariah, frequently belittling me. They often found the most trivial things to pick on me for, like the time I showed up to an open gym with my brand-new SeamCo basketball. The entire time we were at the gym that day they made fun of me for not having a brand-name ball. I never told them my mother got me the ball for my birthday and that, understanding my mother could not afford a brand-name basketball, I was perfectly happy with the SeamCo ball.

Worse than how they treated me themselves was how they reacted when others picked on me. Usually, they joined in on the fun. Perhaps my worst moment in high school occurred the time our cross country team shared a bus to a regional meet with the team from Fairfield's other high school—our arch rival. During the ride home, the guys from our rival school started to taunt me. Even then, my "friends" joined in rather than defend me.

Worst of all, I rarely joined my "friends" on Friday or Saturday nights when they, like most jocks, went out to drink, get high, or just hang out. I wanted to, but they didn't invite me. And that, more than anything else, made me feel ostracized.

Jack stood out as the one guy in this group who came close to being a real friend. Always the last to join in when others taunted me, he also was the first to invite me to join in on an activity. But unlike my friend John in Pittsfield, Jack and I did not become close friends. I never felt comfortable talking to him about the meaning of life and other such issues. Those conversations I had to have with myself.

My Second Family

For all my father's faults, he made a real effort to continue to have a meaningful presence in his children's lives after leaving us to live with Lony. That first summer we visited him regularly at his lake house in Becket, a small town about forty minutes from Pittsfield. However, as the summer drew to a close with my father planning to relocate to Milwaukee and my mother, sisters, and I about to move to Fairfield, I didn't know how often I would see him. This ambiguity gave rise to feelings of angst and confusion. Having gone over and over the events of the past six months, I didn't know what to think or feel about my father. A part of me, still angry at him for leaving me to live with my mother, would have been happy to never see him again. But another part of me knew I needed him. I never addressed these feelings with my father or anyone else.

My father matter-of-factly arranged for us to visit him whenever we had a break from school, as if our visiting him was a foregone conclusion. I have no doubt that in *his* mind it was a foregone conclusion. After all, the normal fears, assumptions, and doubts that most men in his situation likely would have experienced applied to him no more than did the No Entry sign he drove by in the Golan Heights. My mother offered no resistance, and despite whatever feelings my sisters and I had about my father, we were happy for the respite from our mother. So from the beginning of our stay in Fairfield we spent virtually all time we had off from school with him.

For the first year or so, our time with my father was not always entirely pleasant. He never came to Fairfield, except on the rare occasion when he picked us up there to take us to Pittsfield. We always saw him at his place and whenever we saw him, Lony was present. Lony made every effort to get along with us. She was outgoing, energetic, and generally fun to be around. She and Edythe seemed to hit it off immediately. But the tension between Lony, my father, and Mandy could, at times, be palpable.

Lony and my father usually planned at least one or two fun outings for each of our visits. Mandy, however, often refused to go. She had a boyfriend in Pittsfield with a motorcycle, so she could get away whenever she wanted. And, much to my father's and Lony's annoyance, she often did at the most inopportune times, like when we were supposed to be eating dinner together.

My behavior, no doubt, added to the tension. Despite no longer consciously feeling any anger towards Lony, I could not bring myself to talk to her. If she asked me a question, I would answer politely but in as few words as possible. Otherwise, I completely ignored her. I didn't act this way intentionally; it was automatic, like driving a car along a familiar route.

I continued to ignore Lony for well over a year and, to their credit, neither Lony nor my father ever called me on it. Then one day when my cousins, sisters, and I were at the lake house in Pittsfield, my cousin Mitchel noticed my behavior. He took me aside and asked me why I was acting that way. I had no answer. He then told me I was acting like a jerk and should stop. I immediately realized he was right and, from that moment on, I treated Lony like the family member she had become.

Having torn down the barrier that silence had created, I soon discovered Lony shared my sometimes goofy sense of humor. Who would have thought the prim and proper woman I first saw at my father's rental home could belch at will? Edythe and I would tease her about her sometimes slightly off use of English—our favorites were "rollie coaster" and "a dozen of eggs"—and I would pretend to understand Dutch. "Lecker varm," my pronunciation of the Dutch words meaning "nice and warm," came to be our expression for anything good.

During that same visit, I met Lony's kids. My cousin Cliffy and I were watching TV when we noticed a boy about eight years old with light blond hair wandering

around the house looking lost. Curious, we got up, introduced ourselves and asked him if he wanted to watch TV
with us. After a moment of hesitation he joined us and
told us his name was Nathan. A few minutes later, a slightly younger version of Nathan wandered by, saw him, and
also decided to join us. Much less shy than Nathan, Erik
told us his name before even sitting down. We had been
watching TV together for about a half hour when Lony
summoned us to the kitchen for lunch. There I met Liz, a
pretty girl with shoulder length brown hair who looked to
be two to three years older than Nathan. With my father,
Edythe, Mandy, Mitchel, and Cliffy joining us, we had a
pretty big crowd at the table. As we sat down, Lony said
something funny that helped to break the ice. We clicked
almost immediately. Before long, we all were talking and
laughing as if we had known each other forever.

Before long, Lony became like a favorite aunt to me.
We enjoyed joking around. But I was also comfortable
having a serious conversation with her. And at times, she
acted as a buffer between me and my father. As I got older,
my father and I frequently got into heated arguments
about the issues of the day. One argument I remember
well was about whether Jerry Brown, the governor of California and sometimes presidential contender, was a kook
(my father's position) or a politician who should be taken
seriously (my position). Hearing our voices getting louder
and seeing our faces getting redder, Lony intervened, acting as mediator until we both agreed to drop the subject.
Over time, I became much closer to Lony than I was to
my mother. I remained close to Lony long after my father
died and still keep in touch with her.

The best part of the day for me was the time we spent gathered around the dining room table for dinner. We spent almost the entire time laughing. We ribbed each other constantly, but unlike the taunts and put-downs I regularly experienced during school, none of this ribbing was malicious. It was all in good fun. The difference between the nastiness I experienced every time I sat down to dinner at home with my mother and sisters and the love I felt during these dinners could not have been more stark.

Kathy

I couldn't believe my luck when on the first day of the spring semester I saw two beautiful girls seated on either side of me in Expository Writing class. Kathy, a tall, thin, blond with blue eyes, long hair, and legs that seemed to go on forever, sat to my right. Terri, a dark-skinned brunette of average height with big brown eyes, sat on my left. Kathy and Terri were smart, outgoing, and friendly. The three of us became fast friends. We shared lots of laughs, like the time our teacher divided the class into groups of three and gave us thirty minutes to collaborate on an essay about a time of the year. Kathy, Terri, and I wrote a humorous essay we titled "The Daze of Summer." Our essay wasn't very good, but we had lot of fun writing it.

As we got to know each other, I couldn't help noticing Kathy seemed to think many of my remarks were "cute." That and a few wide-eyed looks were all it took for me to fall for her. Having heard her tell me numerous times how much she liked to play tennis, I decided that casually asking her if she wanted to play some time would be the safest way to ask her out. I found it surprisingly easy to do.

And she said yes! We played tennis a few times before I finally found the nerve to ask her out on a real date. Again, she said yes. And so began my first real romance.

A few weeks later I took Kathy to the Junior Prom and there, six months shy of my eighteenth birthday, I had my first real kiss. I stayed with my father in Milwaukee that summer and, before I returned to Fairfield, Kathy broke up with me. But I convinced her to go out with me again the next spring, beginning a close relationship that lasted until halfway through my sophomore year of college.

All the World's a Stage

My mother truly was extraordinarily talented. I didn't appreciate just how talented she was until I saw her act in a play during the summer after my sophomore year of high school. My mother had rejoined the Polka Dot Playhouse and had gotten her first role there in at least eight years. I found out she had gotten the part from hearing her practice through her bedroom door. As I listened to her, I became curious. Since I was a small child I had known she acted. But this was the first time I ever heard her practice and I had never seen her in a play. She clearly had a big part. Remembering how much I struggled to get ready for my Bar Mizvah, I marveled at how she could remember all of her lines.

Then one day, out of the blue, I got a call from one of Mandy's old friends. She wanted to know if I would be interested in going to my mother's play with her. I jumped at the opportunity.

I was not disappointed. My mother's performance blew me away. Her character, not unlike herself, was prone to hysterical outbursts. But unlike at home, her rants were funny. The audience roared with laughter as she yelled her lines. But I didn't laugh. I just sat there, unable to utter a sound as I watched her in awe. A few times her performance seemed so real I feared she might have a heart attack right there on the stage. I gained a whole new appreciation for my mother, but unfortunately the experience did nothing to improve our relationship.

My mother put on a great performance, but she wasn't the only actor on a stage. It seemed everyone I knew spent most of their time playing one role or another. At school almost everybody belonged to one of several well-defined cliques: heads, brains, stage-freaks, gear-heads, do-gooders and, by far the dominant, jocks. I could usually tell, just by looking at someone, what clique he belonged to.

Perhaps because I spent most of my time with the jocks and yet never considered myself a member of their fraternity, their acting was most noticeable—and most distasteful—to me. Very few of them seemed genuine. Most of them seemed intent on shrouding their real selves behind a veil of coolness. They showed off their coolness by bragging about how little time they spent on their school work and by showing not the least bit of interest in the major events of the day. They advertised their apathy, trying their hardest not to be seen trying at anything. I hated the cool kids, not just because I was so un-cool and they picked on me, but because their phoniness was so offensive. I became determined to not be like the cool kids. I would retain my integrity no matter the consequences. I took pride in my un-coolness.

Edythe and I had gotten along reasonably well during our first two years in Fairfield. Sometimes we even had fun together, like when I practiced my Kung Fu moves on her. Then again, that might have been more fun for me than for her. But mostly we continued to live in our separate worlds, rarely paying much attention to each other. She seemed to have lots of friends, but I barely knew them because Edythe rarely hung out with them at our house. I soon realized I barely knew her.

Edythe joined me at Andrew Warde at the beginning of my junior year. Not surprising given the size of the building, our paths rarely crossed during the first few weeks of school. But starting about the middle of October we began to run into each other a little more often—not much more than we had, but enough that I took notice.

Usually I saw her hanging out near the locker rooms with a group of her friends. I walked by quickly, averting my eyes to avoid making contact with any of Edythe's friends. Occasionally, I heard Edythe mutter in a tone of voice I read as embarrassment, "That's my brother," as I sped by.

It took several of these chance encounters, but finally it hit me: Edythe was among the coolest of the cool in the freshman class. I took her coolness as a betrayal. Despite my occasional resentment of Edythe for being both of my parents' favorite she had—until then—been my favorite too. She was, after all, the cute little sister who had put up with my waking her to play Monopoly when I was seven and she was four. She had no idea of how to play the game. But that didn't matter. I moved her token and made decisions for her. I just wanted the company and she was willing to oblige. Although not close, we still got along most of the time.

But to my horror, my cute little sister had grown up to be a charter member of the clique that tormented me daily. I deeply resented her for that. It didn't matter that she had done nothing to earn my wrath. The mere fact that she was part of this clique led me to direct the anger, hurt, and resentment that defined my world at her.

I also had some legitimate reasons for resenting her. Edythe had learned to use her favored status to her advantage and at times could be manipulative. All of the girls in her group of friends were extremely pretty or, to use a more colloquial term, hot. Edythe was quite attractive herself. At first, her friends and I ignored each other. But eventually, perhaps after noticing me staring at one of her friends for a moment too long, Edythe realized she could use their looks to her advantage.

I earned my driver's license in October of junior year, and soon after my mother and I agreed to an unspoken quid pro quo: I took over the responsibility for chauffeuring Edythe around and in turn I occasionally got to use the car myself. At first I didn't mind taking Edythe here and there, but as my resentment grew, her requests began to annoy me. Sometimes, either not wanting to be interrupted or just in a mean-spirited mood, I refused. On a number of occasions, Edythe, unable to get me to change my mind herself, got one of her friends to intervene. Her friend would ask me in her sweetest, sexiest voice if I could please, just this one time, give Edythe a ride. Usually this tactic just made me angry, but every so often it worked. As

I would soon discover, Edythe's attempts to manipulate me were just a warm-up act for what she had in store for my mother.

. . . .

By junior year, my relationship with my mother had reached a sort of negative plateau. We could hardly stay in the same room with each other for more than fifteen or twenty minutes without getting into an argument. So we reached a tacit agreement to spend as little time together as possible. I avoided the kitchen while she made dinner and during weekend mornings when she liked to ease into the day over several cups of coffee, and she, in turn, left me alone after I returned from my evening runs.

Our relationship started its final descent the middle of junior year. It began with my mother's decision to sever her ties with the Polka Dot Playhouse after a falling out with a good friend there. Wanting to remain involved with theater, she answered an ad from Fairfield University's theater program for a volunteer makeup artist. My mother had never done makeup before but, with her artistic talent, found it easy to jump into this role. Always affable around people other than her family, she quickly made new friends there. Flattered to be accepted by this much younger group, my mother began spending a lot of time with them and much less time with her old friends. Before long, my mother's new theater buddies became fixtures at our house. I rarely saw any of her old crowd anymore.

The core group included a cast of characters that could have come from a script by a second-rate playwright. In the lead actress role was Ellen, a bitter, divorced, man-hater and single parent of a three-year old girl. Ellen was in her late thirties. Elaine, an outwardly cheerful woman in her early thirties struggling with loneliness and looking for love in all the wrong places, had the supporting actress role. Gar5y, a self-described "flaming faggot" in his early twenties who was actually a closet heterosexual, had the leading male role. Gar5y happily told anyone who asked that the 5 in his name was silent. The supporting male role went to Rick, a strung-out pothead in his mid-twenties. The remaining characters had bit parts. They included Sheri, an eighteen-year-old Barbie doll blond and high school senior; John, a nineteen-year-old Ken look-alike college freshman and Sheri's boyfriend; and Lisa, a quiet, intelligent woman in her early-twenties. Long after this drama, Lisa and Gary would get married—he had reverted to the more conventional spelling of his name by then.

My mother was forty-five at the time. I had just turned seventeen.

I met Ellen first and this meeting did not go well. Before my mother had even introduced us, Ellen started in on me. "So you're the kid who likes to yell at his mother and call her names," she practically spat at me. I just stood there, flabbergasted, not knowing what to make of this woman. "You think you're smart," she continued, "but you're not smart enough to show your mother some respect."

I felt my cheeks redden but managed to reply in a normal voice, "I don't know who you are and what your problem is, but I don't have to listen to you."

I opened the door and went outside barely able to contain my rage, but not before I heard her say, "Yes, you do have to listen to me and you will."

As I stretched to get ready for my evening run I thought to myself, *Great. As if my mother isn't enough, now I have to deal with this crackpot, too.* My anger propelled me to an exceptionally fast run that evening.

In retrospect, Ellen's timing may have been off, but she had a valid point. When my mother and I argued, I gave as good as I got, frequently calling my mother a bitch, and worse. The only line I made sure never to cross was mentioning her weight. I knew that would have been cruel and, despite my anger, I still felt just enough empathy for her to not go that far.

Within a few days, I met the rest of my mother's friends. She hosted a party for the cast and support crew of a just-finished play to celebrate its success. A crowd of about thirty people filled our living room and spilled into the dining room and kitchen. The smell of pot was hard to ignore as the smoke wafted through the house. Had I not closed my bedroom door, I could easily have gotten high from second-hand smoke. Too many people showed up at this party for me to remember any of their names, but I would soon get to know the main characters well.

This party turned out to be the start of a weekend ritual. Almost every Friday and Saturday night my mother, her core group of friends, and occasionally one or two others congregated in our living room to listen to records, talk, and get high.

These parties really pissed me off. Most of the kids I knew at school who smoked pot worried their parents might find out. And here was my mother partying every Friday and Saturday night with a group that included kids my age. I handled my anger the only way I knew how—by picking fights with my mother. And she responded in kind, often with Ellen by her side, ready to join the attack. The rest knew well enough not to get involved. I became furious at Rick one time when I had a particularly intense argument with my mother and he came to my room to try to calm me down. I seethed as I listened to this dope spew, "Hey, everything is cool man. Relax. Breathe deep and try to slowly let your mind and body reconnect …." and other such blather. Finally, after he suggested I come downstairs and share a joint with my mother, I told him, as politely as I could, "Get the fuck out of my room."

None of the others bothered me. Gary turned out to be a really nice guy. He even took me driving once to help me prepare for the road test I needed to pass to get my driver's license. I liked Elaine. Her bubbly personality made her fun to be around. But when she started joking that she would like to help me give up my virginity, I became a little uncomfortable around her. When she persisted—often to the amusement of my mother—I began to think she might be serious. Unlike the girls in my freshman French class, Elaine never teased or belittled me. I might have taken her up on her offer if not for the fact that I thought she was not very good looking. Not until years later did I realize how inappropriate her advances had been.

. . . .

Meanwhile my relationship with my mother continued its descent. It hit rock bottom when, spurred on by Ellen, she started threatening to kick me out of the house. Believing that any day I might come home to find the locks changed, I considered the logistics of living on my own. The previous summer I had worked forty hours a week washing windows in a hotel at a job my father had arranged. At the end of the summer I bought a 1966 Mustang and put the rest—about $400—into a savings account. Now, with the weather getting warmer every day, I thought maybe I could sleep in my car. I could use Andrew Warde's facilities to shower and brush my teeth. And I would use my savings for food, gas, and other necessities. I had already decided to go to Fordham University, so I had to make this arrangement work only until late August when school would start there.

Fortunately, it never came to that. When I told my father about my predicament he told my mother he would cut her off completely if she went through with her threat. So I stayed, still never completely sure I would be able to get into the house when I got home each day. For the last few months I lived with my mother we were like ghosts, each dead to the other, occupying but not sharing the same house. Not surprisingly, my mother did not attend my high school graduation ceremony. Although her absence did not bother me then, over time it became the one act she committed for which I have never been able to forgive her.

A Fresh Start

It took an innocent question from an acquaintance, Jeff, for me to start thinking about Fairfield as a part of my past. Every day at lunch I sat at the table with my running friends and assorted other jocks and every day I took their abuse. Jeff asked me why I continued to sit with them. Too embarrassed to tell him the truth, I brushed off his question. I had been sitting with my running friends because I didn't want to be seen sitting alone, as if I didn't have any friends. It took Jeff's question for me to accept that the guys I sat with every day were not my friends and I was demeaning myself by sitting with them and taking their verbal bullying.

Along with this acceptance came an epiphany. I would be leaving Fairfield soon, so why should I care what people who would soon be part of my past thought about me? I resolved that from then on I was done with Fairfield. I was done with high school, done with my mother and her friends, and done with Edythe and her shenanigans. I quit the track team and got a job at a restaurant, which often required me to work as late as 1 a.m. on school nights. I slept through most of my classes. And at lunch, I no longer sat with my so-called friends and listened to their insults. I sat by myself wherever I could find an open spot.

About a week later Greg asked me why I had quit track and stopped sitting with him and the other guys at lunch. I replied, in as matter of fact a voice as I could, "I just decided I don't want to sit with you guys anymore pretending you are my friends while putting up with your abuse. I'd rather sit by myself."

He just said "Oh, okay," and walked away with a confused look on his face. I felt a huge weight come off my shoulders as I looked for a place to sit.

Jack, the only person among my running cohorts who had treated me as someone resembling a friend, also planned to go to Fordham. A few weeks after I started sitting by myself at lunch, he asked me if I would be his roommate there. I said no and explained I needed to make a clean break from Fairfield and rooming with him would not allow me to do that. He must have been surprised and hurt, but at the time his feelings didn't even cross my mind. I just wanted to be rid of Fairfield.

Putting high school behind me really lifted my spirits more than I could have imagined. Now, whenever something bad happened, either at home or at school, I would think to myself, *this isn't my life anymore. This is just something I will have to endure for a few more months.* My new perspective paradoxically gave me reason to enjoy, if not savor, my remaining time in Fairfield.

I even made some new friends. Exhausted by late hours working at the restaurant, I often caught up on my sleep during psychology class. But when awake, I had fun goofing off with three of my classmates, Jeff, Andrea, and Joy. I discovered that Jeff, the guy who asked me why I continued to sit with the jocks during lunch, had a quick wit and a great sense of humor. Andrea, a drop-dead gorgeous blond, surprised me by being approachable and friendly. And Joy, who I could always count on to wake me up just before the teacher called on me, possessed the most important quality of all: she laughed at my jokes. Joy also was quite attractive. I probably would have noticed her more had it not been for the dowdy clothes she wore and the fact that she sat next to Andrea. I looked forward to going to psychology class every day. But as much as I enjoyed the daily repartee with Jeff, Andrea, and Joy, I never did anything with any of them outside of psychology class. So when school ended I didn't expect to ever see any of them again.

I continued to experience verbal bullying right up to the last day of school, but, with my new perspective, it no longer had the same impact on me. I often became detached, observing the scene as if not a part of it. Nick, a star on the hockey team and one of the most popular kids at school, regularly picked on me during my Economics class. One day the teacher and a kid who the jocks picked on even more than me—they called him Cheesy—joined in. Rather than get angry this time, I just felt sorry for Cheesy, the teacher, and Nick. I wanted to grab Cheesy by the collar and tell him, "Don't you understand? Nick and his buddies are not your friends and never will be. You may feel better at this moment because they are attacking me and not you, but they will come back to you soon enough. And they'll probably treat you more harshly than ever because you tried to be one of them."

As for the teacher, I thought, *How pitiful that you stoop this low to try to get the class to like you. Any satisfaction from getting the class to laugh with you will be fleeting. You have forfeited any chance you may have had to gain the class's respect.*

But I felt sorriest for Nick. I knew that at eighteen he had already reached the apex of his life. A poor student, a heavy drinker, and the father-to-be of his very pregnant girlfriend's baby, his opportunities were limited. His glory days would end abruptly with graduation.

Strangely enough, my running friends started inviting me out with them on weekends after I stopped sitting with them at lunch. Then they did something I will never forget. They told me I needed to go to the annual sports awards dinner. I told them I had no intention of going. But they insisted. I didn't understand why—I thought they were planning a prank on me. But I finally relented and decided to go. The dinner was an informal affair, held in the school cafeteria. The coach for each sport named the best player on the team, gave a two or three minute speech on how the winner worked hard, showed guts and determination, went to church every Sunday, regularly saluted the American flag, blah, blah, blah.

When Mr. C got up to present the Cross Country award I expected him to name Phil, who regularly finished first for us. Instead I heard him name me as the winner of the Team Effort Award. Confused, I turned around to look at my friends. They signaled by nodding that I had heard correctly. I felt goose bumps as I turned around to listen to Mr. C's speech. I readied myself to soak up the adulation, how I had worked harder than anyone else, how the team had rallied around me to win an important meet—which incidentally would have been our only win of the season— how I went to church every Sunday, despite being a lapsed Jew, blah, blah, blah. But alas, this book is a memoir, not a fantasy or a fairy tale. Mr. C launched into an incomprehensible speech, blathering on for at least 10 minutes without once mentioning me or running. Still, I could feel my heart beat at twice its normal rate as I walked up to accept my trophy. That night my friends took me out drinking with them and I got very drunk.

I got home that night at about 2 a.m. I opened the door and there stood my mother. Her face flushed with anger, she greeted me with a stream of invective.

"Why are you coming home now at two in the morning?" she screamed. "Have you been drinking? Where were you? What am I supposed to think when I have no idea where you are and then you come home this late? I almost called the police."

Normally when my mother yelled at me I instinctively yelled back. But this time, shocked my mother cared enough to worry about where I had been, I waited for her to finish her rant and said, "Sorry, I didn't know you were waiting." Then I went upstairs, brushed my teeth and stumbled into bed, not knowing what to think or feel. Within a few moments I fell into a deep sleep. My mother and I never spoke about that encounter, but it has remained seared in my memory.

The tension at home continued unabated. I spent as much time as I could away from home and, thanks mainly to Kathy, I managed to have a pretty good summer. A few days after graduation, the restaurant where I had been working hired its third head chef in the short time I had been there. He cleaned house, leaving me without a job. But during my brief stay I had learned just enough about cooking to think I could work as a cook. I ended up working a series of jobs, spending enough time at each to keep myself busy and make some pocket change before they discovered my incompetence and fired me.

That summer I played tennis with both Jack and Lou about once a week. But I spent most of my time that summer with Kathy, who I considered to be my only real friend. We played tennis almost every day and, when we couldn't find a court, went to Jennings Beach to work on our tans. I spent far more time at Kathy's house than my own, eating dinner there at least twice a week. Her parents must have approved of me, because they always made me feel comfortable in their home.

Kathy knew exactly what she wanted to do with her life. Since her early teens, she had been passionate about little children. She wanted nothing more than to teach at an elementary school, get married, and have two or three children of her own. Not wanting to move from Fairfield, she hoped one day to teach at Assumption, the Catholic school she attended for nine years. She taught catechism classes there and loved it. Having just completed her freshman year in Western Connecticut State College's Early Education program, Kathy was well on her way toward achieving her goal.

I had no idea what I wanted to do with my life. I just knew I wanted to get away from Fairfield. Had it not been for Kathy, I might never have returned after going away to college…at least not for the next five years.

During my first year of college I came back to Fairfield often to see Kathy. If I needed to stay overnight, I stayed with Mandy, who had transferred from Emerson College to Bridgeport University and lived in a dorm there with her soon-to-be husband Steve. I hoped to never again set foot in the house where I had spent my adolescence. I had no communication with Edythe or my mother and rarely thought about either of them. I had put them in a little room in the back of my mind and shut the door.

During one of my trips late that fall, I saw Edythe as I pulled into a gas station to fill up my tank. All of the bad memories of Fairfield immediately came rushing back. I tried to leave quickly before she had a chance to see me, but had to wait for the car in front of me get out of the way. She saw me and excitedly yelled to her friend, "Hey, that's my brother...that's my brother," as if she had just spotted a rare bird. She came over to my car and, clearly happy to see me, said "Hi, Brother." I don't remember anything either of us said after that, but I knew when I drove away I couldn't continue to hold a grudge against her. We were back to being brother and sister.

Then, during one of my overnight stays the following summer, Mandy told me our mother had sold the house and rented a two bedroom apartment. Mandy asked if I could come to help with the move the following Sunday. My mother's friends all planned to help, Mandy explained, but they could use another strong body. Having already planned to come to Fairfield that weekend to see Kathy, I agreed. My mother and I didn't say a word to each other the entire day but that day marked the beginning of a détente, if not a reconciliation, between us.

CHAPTER 10
FORDHAM

No Boredham at Fordham

So read a headline in our student newspaper, *The Fordham Ram*. It aptly describes one aspect of my college experience, but doesn't begin to tell how rich and rewarding college was for me. I enjoyed the quintessential liberal arts college experience. It is difficult to sum up my time at Fordham without sounding like a marketing brochure. But the fact is, I got everything out of college that a brochure would promise, and more. I took challenging classes that taught me to think critically. I got to know several outstanding professors who took a personal interest in me, including one I remember as a mentor who had a profound impact on my intellectual development. I learned to live with people who had very different values than my own. And I made lasting friendships.

For most of my adult life I have remembered college as a magical time when I made friends easily, got As in most of my classes, and grew from an awkward adolescent to a confident young adult. All this while negotiating only a few minor speed bumps along the way.

I now realize that the time I spent in college was no more four years of uninterrupted bliss than my time in Fairfield was four years of unmitigated hell. Yes, I had many successes in college. But I also endured bouts of depression. I found myself in situations that made me re-think the meaning of tolerance. And I struggled mightily as I tried to understand what made a person good or bad, what constituted success and what role God plays in answering these questions. I am hardly the only person who has dealt with issues such as these in college. But I think the resiliency I developed during my childhood made me better able than many of my peers to prevent the speed bumps from becoming insurmountable obstacles.

. . . .

I had planned to make the seventy-five minute drive from Fairfield to Fordham's Bronx campus by myself on move-in day. But, nervous about finding my dorm and getting information about how the meal plan worked, how to register for classes and so forth, I asked Mandy to join me. Thankfully, she did.

We entered the Rose Hill campus and found our way to Martyr's Court, which would be my home for the next four years. Despite having all the charm of an early-1960s urban renewal project, Martyr's Court had a perfect layout for a newly arrived freshman to quickly make friends. The building comprised six "houses," affectionately called A-house, B-house, and so on. Each house contained eight suites plus two or three single rooms. The suites, which had four bedrooms, a living room and a bathroom, each housed eight students. My room was in suite B-3.

We found my room and there I met the B-house Resident Advisor, Jack. He answered most of my questions and gave me a Welcome Packet that answered the rest. By now I felt I had the situation under control. The first to arrive, I hung out in the living room with Mandy and Jack as my seven new suite-mates trickled in. Mandy's presence had helped to calm me during the drive, but now I couldn't wait for her to leave.

That first night, Fordham put on the best party I had ever attended, providing live music and as much free beer we could drink, since the legal drinking age in New York was eighteen. After the official party ended, we all crossed the trestle over the railroad tracks and headed to the near-by dive bars. Most of the incoming freshman class got wasted that night.

The next day, after rolling out of bed at about eleven with a terrible headache, I went to look for the coach of the cross country team. I knew the scholarship athletes would all be faster than me, but naively thought I could join the team as a walk-on. I found the coach and introduced myself. He greeted me warmly and asked me how fast I had run in high school. I answered proudly that I nearly achieved my goal of running at a sub 6:00-minute a mile pace over my high school's 3.2-mile cross country course. He replied that most of the guys on his team ran about a minute a mile faster over a very hilly five-mile course. He thanked me for my interest and wished me well.

His words did not entirely surprise me. They merely confirmed what I had suspected, but had a major impact on me nevertheless. They forced me to accept for the first time that my competitive running career was over. I had to re-adjust my thinking. I could still think of myself as a runner but running should no longer be the main focus of my life. I resolved right then and there to put all the effort I used to put into running into being the top student in my class. Having discovered that my SAT scores were about a hundred points higher than average for the incoming freshman class, I saw no reason why I couldn't get straight As. I made that my goal.

I went for a long slow run to ponder my decision and then took a nap. After waking up and going to the dining hall for a quick dinner, I went back to B-3 and got ready for another night of uninhibited inebriation with my new friends.

I liked my new suite-mates—they really knew how to party! After the third day of waking up with a hangover, though, I realized I could not keep pace. I was ready to stop. But my suite-mates kept partying on…and on…and on. They began to draw attention on campus for their wild drunken antics. Proud of their growing reputation, six of my suite-mates, plus another guy, Neil, who lived in another suite, called themselves "The Flying Toasters," after the iconic Jefferson Airplane album cover. My roommate got drunk the first twenty-one days—yes, I counted—loudly stumbling into our room at about three each morning.

I realized something had to change. I had become fed up with my roommate's early morning sloshing about our room. I had no interest in becoming a Toaster. I didn't even like the Jefferson Airplane album, which my suite-mates played over and over again. The one other guy in my suite who did not join the Toasters dropped out of school after just two weeks. That clearly was not an option for me. Neither was complaining to our RA.

The solution stared me in the face, but I didn't see it

at first. Neil complained frequently about how his suite-mates were all nerds and geeks. We enjoyed laughing with Neil about them. For a few fleeting moments I thought about the possibility of switching rooms with Neil. But I quickly rejected this idea, too. Despite my suite-mates' late-night carousing I had settled into my home in B-3 and become comfortable there. I didn't want to start all over a month into the school year, especially if it meant rooming with a bunch of nerds. But then, after one too many mornings waking up bleary-eyed, it hit me like a two-by-four. *Who am I fooling?* I said to myself. *I was not "born to be wild." I was "born to be mild." I am a nerd and proud of it. I should embrace the opportunity to room with a suite full of like-minded people.*

I asked Neil if he wanted to switch rooms and he gladly said yes. The dorm director approved and the next day we moved our stuff into each other's room. A little over a month into college I had navigated my way past two speed bumps. Either one might have been a major obstacle had I not had so many opportunities to learn resiliency during my childhood.

The Mind-Body Problem

After a long, Byzantine registration process, classes began—exactly one week and one day after I arrived on campus. Confident I would do well, I also found the prospect of starting at a whole new level of education a little daunting. During high school, my teachers often tried to motivate us to develop good study habits by telling us how much more difficult college work would be and how much less willing our professors would be to put up with our transgressions. Our college professors, my high school teachers warned us, had no tolerance for tardiness, talking in class, or turning in assignments late. The college professors in these stories always seemed to have a plane to catch. If we didn't turn our paper in on time, we were warned, our professor would not have it with him when he flew off to wherever professors went to grade papers, and we would get zero credit.

I had taken two Advanced Placement (AP) classes in high school, Modern European History and Calculus, and had to work harder than I ever had before just to keep up. Now I would be taking four college level classes. I braced myself for the hard work ahead.

But I found my first semester freshman classes at Fordham easy—much easier than the AP classes I had taken in high school. This was especially true for Calculus. I had struggled with the more abstract, theoretical topics in high school—the first time I ever had difficulty in math—and decided to take calculus again in college in the hope I would gain mastery of the subject. But the college version of calculus did not include any of the proofs and theorems that had bedeviled me the first time around.

I breezed through Calculus, English Composition and Intro to Microeconomics. Ironically, the only class that challenged me was French, the same subject I had struggled with during freshman year in high school. But unlike my French teacher in high school, who mocked me in front of the class for being so ill-prepared, my French professor at Fordham was an outstanding teacher. I spent twice as much time studying and doing homework for this class as for all three of my other classes combined. I might not have worked quite so hard had I been willing to settle for a B, but I was hell-bent on getting straight As. I ended the semester with three As and a B+, the B+ in French.

I began to think I was smarter than my classmates. I even became a little frustrated with what I saw as my professors' penchant for teaching to the slowest students in the class. But in retrospect, I realize I was not necessarily smarter than anyone else. I was just better prepared—the exhortations of my high school teachers had had their desired effect.

Roughly two-thirds of the students in my freshman class commuted. The commuters, by and large, had attended high schools that did not have a college track. Many of these students were the first in their families to attend college and the majority of them worked while attending school. They had a much higher freshman dropout rate than the borders (as we called those of us who lived on campus.) Some of the entry-level classes may have been taught at a slower pace to give commuters a chance to acculturate to college-level work.

Meanwhile, I enjoyed what was for me a rich social life. Most weekends I went back to Fairfield to be with Kathy. She rarely came to Fordham. I usually left for Fairfield on Saturday morning and returned late Sunday night, staying with Mandy at University of Bridgeport on Saturday nights. Officially, Mandy shared a standard-issue college dorm room in a high-rise building on campus, but she actually lived with the dorm director in his relatively spacious apartment in the same building. Steve, whom Mandy married a couple of years later, rarely said anything to me. Wearing a tank top, shorts, and three-day-old beard, he never looked pleased to see me when I arrived, usually at about one in the morning. Still, I was happy to have a place to crash—my mother's house would have been far more convenient, but that was not an option.

My life had improved dramatically—not just because of the new friends I had made, but also because of the old tormentors I left behind. I no longer had to listen to my mother's tirades or worry about her kicking me out of the house. And I no longer had to endure the taunts and insults of the bullies in school. There was no cool or un-cool at Fordham. I could be myself and not worry about the repercussions. Without even thinking about it, the pain and humiliation I had suffered during my childhood and adolescent years started to recede into the depths of memory.

When reminiscing about school, people often recall the one great teacher who had a major impact on their lives. For me that was Dr. Paul Fitzgerald. He taught the introductory philosophy class, The Mind-Body Problem, which I took my second semester at Fordham. I signed up for his class mainly to begin satisfying the Fordham requirement to take a combination of five philosophy and theology classes. But the title of the class also intrigued me. What was the mind-body problem?

Dr. Fitzgerald must have had a reputation as an espe-cially difficult teacher because only three other people took his class with me. On the first day he told us the class would be an inquiry into the age-old conundrum,

"Are our minds inexorably linked to our bodies?" or put another way, "Do people have souls that live on after they die?" The implications of this question, he told us, are profound. Most, if not all, major religions assume the answer to this question is an emphatic yes. But how do we know? Can we ever know?

I had wondered about questions such as these since, as a twelve-year-old, I began to doubt much of what I had learned during my Jewish upbringing. But this was not a topic I felt comfortable talking about with others. To my peers these questions were irrelevant and stupid. To my parents and teachers they were at best inappropriate and annoying and at worst blasphemous.

Dr. Fitzgerald approached the mind-body problem in a strictly analytical way, using logic and deductive reasoning to gain insights. He taught the class using the Socratic method, asking questions of us and challenging our assumptions until we reached a truth relevant to our inquiry. This way of thinking was a revelation. I wish I could remember some of the specific analytical paths he took us down with his questioning. But these are less important than the process he used to take us down these paths. His rational approach validated my questioning about God and religion as a worthwhile intellectual endeavor. I felt liberated in his classroom.

More than any other teacher I had before, Dr. Fitzgerald taught me how to think critically. He encouraged his students to challenge conventional wisdom, including what he taught us. At times he could be intimidating. I vividly recall one incident when he asked a student a question about some material we had covered during the previous class. The student spouted back—almost word for word—what Dr. Fitzgerald had told us. Dr. Fitzgerald then moved to an empty seat right next to his hapless victim and asked, "Do you really believe that crap they teach you in college?" He wanted the student to either defend the logic of the argument from the previous class or challenge it—not to simply accept and memorize it.

I was chomping at the bit as my classmate suffered through Dr. Fitzgerald's interrogation. I saw a flaw in his logic from the previous day and I want to tell him about it. For me, Dr. Fitzgerald's Mind Body class became like a game of chess. He would advance a position and I would come back the next class ready to challenge it. If I didn't get a chance during class I asked to talk to him afterword. He seemed to have unlimited time to talk with me and appeared to enjoy the verbal sparring as much as I did.

I got straight As the spring semester of my freshman year and was admitted to Fordham's Honors Program. I had told only one or two students about my grades, but when I returned for my sophomore year everyone seemed to know. People treated me with a measure of respect and admiration I hadn't known before. At Fordham, I discovered, it was cool to be smart. My self-confidence grew exponentially. In a little over a year I had changed the way people perceived me as well as how I looked at myself.

Marathon Man

During high school, it seemed that most of the strangers I passed by as I ran looked at me as if belonged to slightly eccentric cult. But by the start of my junior year of college, 1978, running had become a major fad. Now it seemed that almost everybody wanted to join in. And non-runners seemed genuinely interested in understanding why someone would want to run just for the sake of running. *The Complete Book of Running* by Jim Fixx was a best seller that year. No longer an eccentric, I felt vindicated.

The New York City Marathon had become a major event by 1978, having the year before changed its route to cover all five boroughs of the city. Since the previous spring, I had been thinking about trying to live out my high school dream of running a marathon. Finally in August I decided to go for it.

With the marathon scheduled for Sunday, October 22, I had two months to get ready. I started my training already in excellent shape, having had plenty of time that summer as a camp counselor to go for long runs. To say I trained would be a gross overstatement. I really had no idea of how to train for a marathon. I just gradually increased the length of my long runs until I could comfortably run sixteen miles.

As race day approached, I got myself into a cycle of running long and hard every fourth day. The Thursday before the marathon I cruised effortlessly at a very fast pace for sixteen miles. I was ready. I planned to run the first sixteen miles just slightly slower than a pace I felt I could maintain for 26.2 miles and then, if I felt good, I would run as hard as I could for the rest of the race. Not coincidentally, the sixteenth mile mark came just before turning on to First Avenue, after crossing the Fifty-ninth Street Bridge. My father and Lony lived at Sixty-fourth and Second Avenue at the time, so I knew they would be there to cheer me on.

Had I known anything about training for and running a marathon I would have realized that I had concocted a hare-brained strategy. But it worked. The race could not possibly have gone better. I reached the 16-mile mark in exactly two hours feeling like I had just done a warm up jog. I took off as planned and immediately started flying by people. When I turned onto First Avenue about a quarter mile later, a wall of people greeted me and the other runners, cheering us on. I hadn't expected that. I also hadn't expected Lony to cue the people around her to cheer for me as I went by. When I heard a throng of people scream "Go Ira" I felt like I was running on a cushion of air, although I did come down to earth a little after hearing someone mutter under his breath, "Who the hell is Ira?"

I continued to run effortlessly up First Avenue, gliding by the other marathoners and soaking in the cheers from the crowd. After I crossed the bridge into the Bronx, I yelled out to the crowd, "The Bronx is the best," and they responded with a resounding cheer. I didn't start to feel tired until about the twenty-third mile, and even then it felt nothing like the dreaded Wall I had heard so much about. I finished in 3:05, which meant I had run the last ten miles at a 6:30 per mile pace. I came in 1,025th place out of 8,588 finishers (7,819 males) who completed the race.

I came back to campus that evening a minor celebrity. (I might have been a bigger celebrity had my roommate, Dave, not also run the race. Dave, the star of Fordham's cross country and track teams, finished in 2:24 and came in twenty-ninth place overall.) People I barely knew came up to congratulate me and ask about the race. The editor of *The Fordham Ram*, Neal, asked me to write an article describing my experience. The self-confidence I got from running soared to a whole new level. I now believed I could accomplish anything.

I never did get an article published in *The Fordham Ram*, though. Writing had never come easily for me; instead of just recounting my experience running the marathon I angst-ed over how to make the article interesting to non-runners. After several attempts and many hours I gave up and went back to my school work. Embarrassed by my inability to write the article, I made a point to avoid Neal whenever I saw him for the next several weeks.

I ran the NYC Marathon again the next year, but this time with different results. I had stayed up most of Thursday night into the Friday morning before the race working on a paper. I woke up Sunday morning still feeling the after-effects of my near-all-nighter. And to make matters worse, the weather forecast for the day was hot, sunny, and humid, the worst possible conditions for running a marathon.

Despite starting out slowly I began struggling at about the ten-mile mark. A few times I poured water over my head and I could actually feel the water simmer, as if I had poured it into a hot frying pan. By the time I reached the half-way point I knew I wasn't going to finish. I just wanted to make it to First Avenue and Sixty-fourth Street so I could go to my father's apartment, take a shower and get some sleep. As I turned onto First Avenue, I heard the roar of the crowd, but this time the noise only added to my misery. Any remaining doubt I had about whether I should stop was erased at about Sixty-first Street. Both calves cramped up, one a few seconds after the other. I stood, literally stuck in the middle of the street, unable to move until the cramps subsided. I walked the rest of the way to Sixty-fourth Street, where I saw my father and Lony and got off the course.

My father couldn't hide his disappointment. But even as we walked to his apartment, I had already accepted what happened and was ready to move on. I had simply encountered a bad set of circumstances that had combined to make it a bad day for me. Fortunately, the novelty of running a marathon had passed, so when I got back to campus this time nobody seemed to care all that much about how I did.

The Man with a Future

My suite-mates traded insults with each other as if it were a sport. Until about midway through my sophomore year I felt I was on the receiving end of more than my fair share. It was mostly in good fun, though—never nearly as bad as in high school. Each semester, it seemed, my confidence grew and people respected me more. I took classes with all the toughest professors and still got straight As. I finished with a 3.94 GPA.

When I was accepted into Northwestern's PhD program in Economics, my suite-mate Jim started calling me "The Man with a Future." And truly I was. Had there been a vote among my friends for Most Likely to Succeed, I would have won unanimously.

But the demons from my childhood still lurked somewhere in the recesses of my memory.

CHAPTER 11
ARE YOU GOING TO SAN FRANCISCO

I began my adventure in San Francisco two days after graduating from Fordham. I wanted to get as far away from home as possible. I needed to prove to myself I could make it on my own, even if only for the summer. And I had come to love San Francisco after having spent the last two college spring breaks there. I couldn't get over how much more livable and beautiful San Francisco was compared to New York City—I enjoyed telling people how if you ran in Central Park as far as you could go in one direction you ended up in Harlem. But if you ran in Golden Gate Park as far as you could go in one direction you reached the Pacific Ocean.

Still, the decision to spend the summer in San Francisco had not been easy. I faced a dilemma that made me the envy of some of my friends, but forced me to make one of the most difficult decisions of my life. Kathy and I had parted company sophomore year. By senior year, I had two incredible girlfriends, Mary and Christy, and had to choose between the two. Although far from ready for marriage at the time, I thought it not unlikely I would eventually marry one of them. I couldn't imagine where or how I would ever meet anyone like either of them again.

I hid nothing. I told both Mary and Christy I was not ready to make a lasting commitment. Both agreed we could see other people as long as we were honest with each other. Neither seemed to mind when I told them about the other. This understanding worked in large part because Mary and Christy lived at opposite ends of the continent—Mary in New York and Christy in San Francisco.

I met Christy near the end of my junior year and her senior year, at one of the frequent mixers on campus. We talked for a while and then, wanting to escape the noise, continued our conversation while walking around campus. By the end of our walk, perhaps three hours later, I was completely taken with her. With only four weeks to go before Christy's graduation, we savored every moment we had together. Then she went back home to San Francisco.

Christy and I stayed in close contact by exchanging letters and occasionally talking on the phone. Then, almost six months since the last time we had seen each other, she called to give me some wonderful news. She would be coming to New York for a few days in November for her sister Jackie's wedding. Christy invited me to attend the wedding as her special guest. At the wedding I reacquainted myself with Jackie and her groom Patsy, both of whom had also gone to Fordham. I also met Christy's parents and brother, Tom. Christy's parents made me feel as if I too had just become a part of their family, and Tom and I started a friendship that would become as close as any I had up to that point in my life, including with Christy. The love I felt from Christy's entire family took me off guard. I had never experienced anything like it before. It became stronger still when I went to San Francisco the following March during spring break to visit Christy and her family.

My relationship with Mary was more complicated. We met in an ancient philosophy class during the fall semester of my sophomore year. Her long red hair, green eyes, and curves-in-all-the-right-places body caught my attention the first day of class. After a few classes, I also noticed her intelligence—unlike me, she seemed to understand our professor's stream-of-consciousness lectures.

I knew I had to ask Mary out. This time I needed only a few weeks to muster the courage. I asked her if she might be interested in going with me to see a special Christmas exhibit at The Museum of Natural History. She said yes, no doubt expecting that after the museum we would head back to the Bronx. But I had bigger plans. After the museum, I took her first to dinner at the Magic Pan, an inexpensive but very nice restaurant, and then to another restaurant known for its desserts. We had a great time. She later told me she marveled at how meticulously I had planned the date, but so matter-of-factly suggested we go from one place to the next. But when we got to her apartment Mary told me she was twenty-four years old—I had just turned twenty—and had recently experienced a painful end to a close relationship. She added that she was not ready to get into another. She offered to be "just friends." Although disappointed, I took her at her word and gladly accepted the offer.

Mary and I soon became close friends. But our relationship was not one of equals. I worshipped her. Mary possessed beauty, intelligence, worldliness, and spirituality unlike anybody I had ever met before. I felt honored that someone like her would actually take an interest in me, just as I did as a ten-year-old when my high-school-aged neighbor Paul asked me to go fishing with him. For her part, Mary told me she liked me for my thoughtfulness, determination, and lack of guile.

A philosophy and theology double major, Mary shared my new-found interest in philosophy. We had many deep conversations about Plato, Aristotle, and the other philosophers we studied in class. More often than not, these conversations veered into discussions about religion, God, and the meaning of life. Mary, a devout Catholic, seemed to have it all figured out. But I continued to struggle with fundamental questions like whether God existed and, if so, whether he paid any attention to me. I considered myself to be an ethical person, but without religion, I lacked a clear moral compass to guide me. Mary prayed for my soul.

Over time, as I revealed more and more of my past, Mary came to appreciate me for my resiliency. At the same time, she became a sort of life mentor to me. More than any teacher, friend or coach, and certainly more than either of my parents, she gave me the confidence to finally feel good about myself. I often confided in her when I doubted myself or suffered one of my frequent bouts of depression. Mary would tell me how special I was, usually lifting me out of my funk.

However, much to my frustration, Mary would not have a romantic relationship with me. I chased her for nearly two and a half years. Finally, just weeks before my graduation, after we shared a couple of bottles of wine over dinner in her apartment, she said, "Ira, the ball is your court." How could I say no?

As graduation approached, I struggled with my decision. Finally, Mary made it for me. She told me she understood how much I wanted to get away from New York and that she did not want me to resent her for not taking the opportunity to go to San Francisco. I think she also knew something I had only begun to sense: as much as we admired and respected each other, we did not love each other as romantic partners. We agreed to remain friends, but put our romantic relationship on hold for the next few months and then decide how we felt about each other.

. . . .

My summer in San Francisco started well enough. My first full day there I went to the University of San Francisco housing office to see if I could find an ad for a sublet. Christy and Tom had offered to let me stay with them but I needed to venture out on my own. I found several ads and by the end of the day had signed a sublet agreement for a room in a very nice apartment just three blocks from Golden Gate Park—perfect for running. The sublet cost a fraction of what I had expected to pay but my room came unfurnished. I fixed this problem by buying an inexpensive futon to use as a bed and getting milk crates from a nearby grocery store to use as a dresser and night table.

The next day I assigned myself the task of finding a job. Early that morning I picked up a copy of *The San Francisco Examiner*, turned to the Help Wanted section and circled the ads for the jobs I thought I might have a chance of getting. Then I started calling. In less than an hour I scored an interview with Otis Spunkmeyer Old Tyme Burritos for later that afternoon. They planned to open a new store downtown and needed people to manage it. Twenty minutes into the interview they offered me a job as assistant manager. Having enjoyed my experience managing the Planter's Snack Shoppe in Wildwood, New Jersey, the previous summer, I took the job, despite a salary offer only 50 cents above minimum wage.

I could not have been more proud of myself. In just two days I had found a place to live, furnished it, and found a job. I basked in my accomplishment, not realizing those two days would turn out to be the highlight of my summer.

Had I not been so busy proving I could make it on my own I might have noticed sooner that Christy harbored some resentment toward me. Her warm embrace at the airport belied a simmering anger that lay just beneath the surface. Clueless at first, I began to suspect something might be wrong after about a week. Christy appeared to be holding back; at times she seemed almost aloof. I found it difficult to engage her in conversation. Between doing her household chores, catching up with her brother Tom on his day off, and hanging out with a friend of theirs who lived in the apartment across the hall, Christy rarely seemed to have time to be alone with me. Although frustrated, I didn't say anything about it because I was unsure whether my impressions were valid.

I found myself spending much more time than I had expected at my new job. A young, fast-growing company, Otis Spunkmeyer had gained traction in California with its Olde Tyme Cookies. The Olde Tyme Burrito store they had hired me to help manage was the pilot for what they hoped would be a second successful line of business.

I worked sixty-plus hours during each of my first two weeks, helping the district manager and corporate staff prepare for the Grand Opening. In the process, I missed several outings Christy had planned. The long hours continued after the store opened as my bosses struggled to hire and train a stable cadre of workers.

Just days after the store opened my immediate supervisor, the store manager, quit. The next day, the district manager offered me the manager position. I told him I would take it if he would give me either Saturday or Sunday off each week. I also asked if I could have both days off the weekend after next so I could join Christy and her family on a long-planned trip to Yosemite. My boss said he really needed me to work both days the upcoming weekend, but after that would try his best to accommodate me. I accepted the promotion. The following Thursday I reminded my boss that I needed the weekend off. Much to my surprise, he responded by telling me he didn't think that would be possible.

I realized then I had made a mistake. Christy worked Monday through Friday—when would I ever get to see her if I had to work on weekends? I simply could not miss the trip to Yosemite. I came to work the next day, worked my shift, and then quit.

Christy, Tom, and I drove to their parents' house near Sacramento and early the next morning we packed into the car and headed for Yosemite. I detected not a hint of resentment from Christy's parents. They made me feel so welcome and at ease that at times I actually found it a little unsettling. I was far from ready to make a long-term commitment to Christy and yet they treated me as if I were already part of their family.

I spent most of the weekend in Yosemite hiking with Tom, while Christy all but ignored me. Finally, my frustration near the boiling point, I confronted her. She admitted she had been keeping me at a distance. Then she told me it really wasn't okay for me to have a relationship with Mary. I reacted with anger. "Why didn't you tell me that before I came out to San Francisco?" I asked. I felt she had lured me to San Francisco under false pretenses. I had been completely open and honest with her. And she had responded with inviting letters, urging me to spend the summer with her.

Christy had good reason to feel resentment toward me, though. Yes, I had been open and honest with her. But she had waited patiently for almost an entire year only to have me tell her just weeks before beginning our summer together that I had a relationship with Mary. To make matters worse, I had previously told Christy how I had idolized Mary. We rode back first to Sacramento and then to San Francisco in stony silence.

The rest of the summer we went through the same cycle over and over again. I would ask Christy to spend more time with me, then she would tell me, usually indirectly, I needed to choose between her and Mary and I would refuse. Around and around we went.

That August I received a letter from Mary telling me she had become very close to another guy. After reading her letter I felt more relief than disappointment: we could now go back to being friends. Mary and I kept in touch for years afterwards.

The Monday after returning from Yosemite I set out to find a new job. This time I only considered positions that didn't involve weekend work. Having found a job so easily the first time, I thought I would find something quickly. I didn't. Every morning I picked up *The San Francisco Examiner*, circled the jobs I thought I had a chance of getting, and started calling. I also looked up job placement agencies in the Yellow Pages and called several of them. I got two or three interviews a week.

Most of the people who interviewed me realized immediately upon looking at my resume that I was over-qualified. They didn't believe my lie that I planned to stay in San Francisco indefinitely. Along the way Radio Shack offered me a job as a store manager. I turned it down when I learned they expected me to spend the first three months in their training program for new store managers. Lying about how long I would stay in a job I could learn in a day or two didn't seem so bad, but letting a company invest in me for the two and a half months I had left in San Francisco would have been over the line.

I also got a second interview for a financial analyst job at one of the big San Francisco banks. I couldn't believe my luck when this opportunity came up. I thought I might have stumbled on a solution to the problems that had been vexing me all summer. Since receiving Northwestern's acceptance letter I had been unsure whether an economics PhD program was the right career choice for me. I had chosen this path not because I had a passion for economics, but because I thought I would do well—at Fordham I had earned a B+ in one economics class and As in the rest while expending a minimal amount of effort—and I couldn't think of anything else to do. The bank job paid

well and would look good on my resume. Equally important, taking the job would demonstrate my commitment
to Christy and give us time to decide whether we were
right for each other. I reasoned I could defer my acceptance to Northwestern for a year and decide then whether
I still wanted to go there. I made my decision; I would take
the job and stay in San Francisco. All I had to do now was
get the offer.

By the day of the interview I had convinced myself the
job was not only my best choice, it was my only choice. I
had wrapped myself up into a ball of anxiety. Not surprisingly, the interview did not go well. I could almost feel my
forehead blinking in bright red letters "Too Nervous." The
man interviewing me saw the sign as clearly as I felt it. I
didn't get the position.

I returned to my job search, numbly repeating the now
familiar routine of checking the help wanted pages and
making phone calls each morning. I became morose. Each
day, I lost a little more self-confidence. I missed my friends
from Fordham. I began to feel isolated and lonely. The
warmth and affection from Christy, Tom, and their parents reminded me how distant I felt from my own family.

Edythe came out to San Francisco that summer—by
then we had long since reconciled—and stayed with me
for a couple of weeks before moving in with her friends.
Her visit lifted my spirits a little, but the effect was fleeting. My father and Lony also visited the city for a couple
of days. While they were in town, they took Christy and
me to dinner. After dinner, Christy remarked that she felt
the long-standing tension between my father and me that
I had told her about. His visit deepened my mood.

152

I slogged on with my job search until finally, almost six weeks after the trip to Yosemite, I responded to an ad from a collection agency that appeared regularly in the help wanted pages. I got through to Mr. Michaels on the first try. Ignoring the normal niceties, he launched right into the interview, belligerently firing questions at me. Pissed off about my situation and not really wanting to work in a collection agency, I responded in an equally belligerent manner. He had hoped I would respond that way. He offered me the job and asked me to start the next day. I reluctantly accepted.

Located in Sunnyvale, a charmless suburb about thirty miles south of San Francisco, the call center was a two hour ride from my apartment on two different buses. The workplace consisted of a large open space with about thirty desks facing a white board with tallies of each agent's weekly collections, a private office for the general manager, and a small conference room. Mr. Michaels—a fake name—led me to the conference room, where I joined two other people starting that day. There I learned our job was to find debtors and intimidate them into paying up. The company had prepared "talk-offs," which Mr. Michaels told us to use as our opening salvos. We spent the rest of the day doing role plays.

The following day Mr. Michaels assigned us each a desk with a drawer full of files on our book of debtors. He strongly recommended we use aliases for our personal safety. I chose David Friedman. The atmosphere in the office was highly competitive and nasty. Whenever someone made a large collection he would yell out how much he had just collected, let out a few whoops, and run to the whiteboard to proclaim his victory. At least a couple of times a day someone made a display of loudly shouting threats at a debtor before ending the call by slamming his phone down. The office erupted in cheers after these outbursts.

During lunch with one of the guys who started with me, I learned he lived just a couple of blocks off my bus route. I asked if I could ride with him and he agreed, thereby shortening my commute by forty-five minutes each way. This arrangement worked well until one day near the end of the summer Mr. Michaels changed the shift assignments. My car pool buddy and I were assigned different shifts, meaning I now had a two-hour-each-way multiple-bus commute again. I asked Mr. Michaels if he could please keep my friend and me on the same shift. Before Mr. Michaels could answer, another guy who frequently needled me for my somewhat gentler approach to collecting intervened. He said loudly enough for everyone to hear, "Stop being such a baby. Just take whatever shift you're assigned." I flew into a rage, shouting "Mind your own fucking business" and got out of my chair ready to fight. My tormentor cowered back into his seat. The rest of the office met my explosion with silence and disbelief. I was as surprised as anyone, and deeply embarrassed. At the end of the day Mr. Michael assured me I would remain on the same shift as Ted. He also praised me for my outburst and said he would like to see more of that from me. Three weeks later, a couple of days after bringing in a huge payment using my gentler approach, I quit.

Meanwhile the strain in my relationship with Christy continued. I thought our relationship had remained on an even keel, not improving but not getting any worse. Then on August 29, two days before my lease was to run out,

Christy broke up with me. I was devastated. I told her I would try to get a ticket to New York and stay there until school started at Northwestern. But she and Tom asked me to stay with them until September 17, as planned. Hoping I could somehow repair my relationship with Christy, I agreed to stay. The weekend before I left for Chicago, we went back to Yosemite with Tom and their parents. This time I all but ignored Christy. I needed the time to myself. On our way home, we stopped to take a look back at the park. The view was amazing. I stood alone at first, but then Christy came up beside me and took my hand. Three days later I sat in a plane watching San Francisco fade into the distance. I wondered what the next destination would bring.

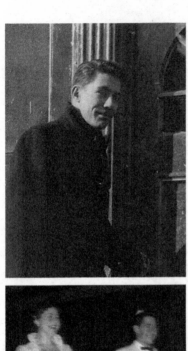
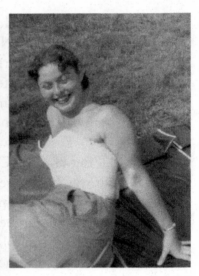
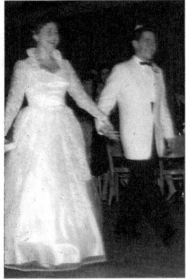

Top left: My father, a man of mystery and intrigue

Top right: My mother, the pin-up girl

Center left: Albert and Annette, the happy, beautiful couple

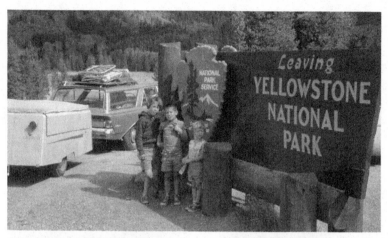

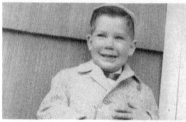

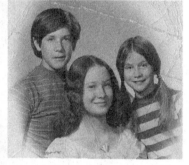

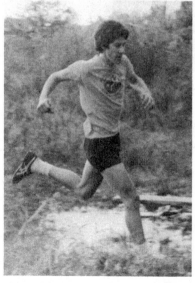

Top: My sisters and me at Yellowstone National Park, circa 1965

Center left: This picture was just too cute not to include

Center right: Me, with my sisters Mandy and Edythe, in the passport photo for our trip to Israel

Bottom left: Running a high school cross country race against our school's arch rival

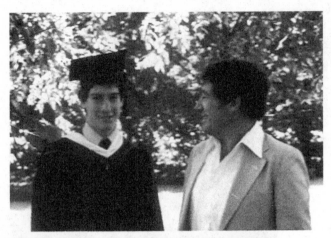

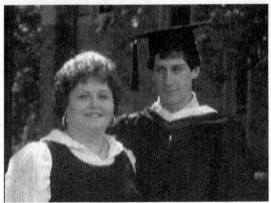

Top: My father congratulating me at my graduation from Fordham

Bottom: While my mother boycotted my high school graduation, she did attend my college graduation

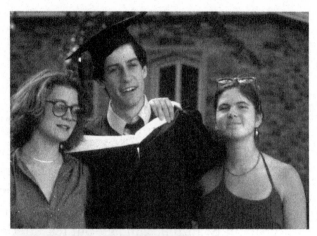

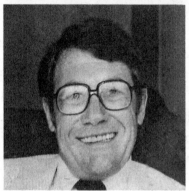

Top: Me, with Edythe and my stepsister Elizabeth

Bottom: My father, the vibrant executive
I remember best

CHAPTER 12
EVANSTON OR BUST

September 17, 1980. I looked out the window and watched the city fade away as the plane gained altitude. I knew exactly where I was going—to Engelhart Hall, a dorm for graduate students at Northwestern University in Evanston, Illinois—but felt utterly lost.

A Foreign Land

I continued to look out the window until after we passed over the Sierra mountain range and the view became uninteresting. I tried to read, but the words had no meaning. My mind kept drifting back to Christy. I tried to understand what went wrong as I relived scenes with her over and over again in my mind. But I couldn't find an answer. I knew only that our relationship, like a cracked egg, could not be put back together again.

The pilot woke me from my reverie when he announced our initial descent into O'Hare. I looked out the window again and saw a landscape that looked completely foreign to me—flat in every direction as far as I could see. The "Welcome to Chicagoland" sign at the end of the long walk through the terminal made me feel even more like a stranger in a foreign land. Chicagoland? *What am I doing here?* I asked myself.

I retrieved my bags from the carousel and with considerable effort managed to get a duffel bag on my back, an enormous suitcase in one hand, and two smaller bags in my other hand. I do not recall what I put in each, but I have no doubt I packed inefficiently. I looked for a help desk, but could not find one, so I resorted to asking anyone I saw in a uniform where I could catch the Evanston bus. None of them knew. Finally, I saw a portly policeman standing next to the glass door that opened up to Chicagoland.

I asked, "Can I ask you a question?"

He replied, laughing, "You just did."

But then, taking pity, he showed me where to go to wait for the Evanston bus. Carrying almost all my earthly possession in four bags, I inched my way to the bus stop, wondering what the rest of the people in *Chicagoland* must be like if the airport cops were such wise-asses.

After what seemed like an eternity, the bus that would take me to my new home arrived. I sat down in the nearest window seat hoping to see something interesting, but mile after mile, the view was the same. Exhausted by the long plane ride, endless taxi-ing around the tarmac, and carrying my four bags to the bus stop, I nodded off. I awoke with a jolt when I heard the bus driver bark, "Evanston. Next and last stop." I would have to complete the last leg of my journey, about three quarters of a mile, on foot. Lugging my bags, which together must have easily weighed over a hundred pounds, I slowly made my way to Englehart Hall, taking frequent rest stops along the way. (In 1980, roller bags were still a curiosity.)

I went to a small office on the first floor and saw a letter taped to the window, saying "Move-in hours begin at 9 a.m. and end at 5 p.m. sharp. Students arriving after 5:00 can pick up their keys at the Department of Public Safety."

Then I looked at my watch. *This can't be true,* I screamed to myself in a rage of self-pity. I fumbled through my bags to find my communications from Northwestern. And there it was—the same letter that was taped to the door.

Too tired to carry my bags another step, I left them at the door and headed out to get my key. Along the way, as I passed some buildings that looked like dorms, I heard what sounded like a tribal chant. Curious and a little apprehensive, I walked toward the sound; when I got close I realized the chant was part of a fraternity rush. Social fraternities did not exist at Fordham, so this was an entirely new experience. My feeling of having landed in a foreign land became stronger still.

I continued on my way to the Public Safety Office without further incident. The officer gave me my keys and a ride to Englehart. I took the elevator up to the third floor, the doors opened, and panic immediately set in. Where were my bags? My hand shaking, it took several tries before I could open the door. I entered to find an apartment with two decent-sized bedrooms, a bathroom, a tiny kitchen, and a space between the doors to the bedrooms just large enough to fit a table and two chairs. The door to the bedroom on the right was closed. I entered the bedroom on the left and found all four of my bags, intact, lying on the floor. Relieved, I suddenly realized how hungry I was, so I went out to get some food.

Upon returning, I opened the door to find a guy with long hair, a full beard, and ragged jeans sitting at the table.

He looked more like a Hell's Angels disciple than a graduate student at an elite university. My new roommate got up and introduced himself. Jim told me he had put the bags in my room because he didn't think they were safe sitting out in the hallway. He hoped I didn't mind. After exchanging a few pleasantries, we started talking about how each of us had ended up at Northwestern and what we came there to study. Jim told me he had come to get a PhD in Organizational Behavior. Five years older than me, he had taken a circuitous route to get there. He had earned Masters degrees from Columbia and the University of Chicago and in between had held jobs as a case worker deciding disability insurance claims for the State of New York and as a construction hand, mostly in his hometown near Albany. He drove a bus for the City of Chicago before starting at Northwestern.

Before we got too far into our conversation, Jim let on he was a huge baseball fan and an avid runner. Jim seemed like a decent guy, although he had a huge black mark against him—he was a Yankees fan. Before heading to our respective rooms to go to sleep, we agreed to go running together the next day.

The next morning, I attended an orientation session for first-year PhD economics students. After welcoming us, the Graduate Student Affairs Chairman for the Economics Department, Dr. B, went over key elements of the program for first year students. He explained the program consisted of three core classes: macro-economics, micro-economics and statistics. These classes were mandatory. In addition, we were strongly encouraged, but not required, to take one elective each quarter; we could take the elective from any department in the graduate school.

Next he explained how the grading worked. He told us we should expect a mandatory weekly homework assignment from each class, which would account for a portion of our grade, and our performance on the midterm and final exams would account for the rest. He recommended that we form study groups to work together on the homework assignments.

I noticed a slight grin on his face before he turned to the next topic. He told us not to be alarmed when we received the scores from our first exam. Clearly enjoying the confused looks on our faces, he went on to explain that the economics department graded on a curve and they designed their tests to result in a normal distribution around a median score of about sixty. That meant someone scoring a sixty on a test could expect to find himself in the middle of the pack. He explained further that what mattered was not our individual performance but how we performed relative to our classmates. In other words, we would compete with the same people with whom we would spend most of the day in class and with whom we were encouraged to collaborate on our homework assignments.

It took a couple of weeks for the next surprise to sink in. The chairman of the economics department at Fordham had told me to expect a mathematical orientation in my graduate program. At his suggestion, I had taken a graduate level course he taught, called Math for Economists. I had sailed through the class, acing it with minimal effort. I thought I was prepared for the PhD curriculum at Northwestern.

But a day or two later I learned the three core courses required an understanding of Real Analysis. Despite its rather prosaic name, Real Analysis is a highly abstract and, to my mind, extremely difficult subject. According to Wikipedia, it "… is typically taken in college after a two- or three-semester course in calculus, and usually after a course in rigorous mathematical proof." I had taken a two-semester calculus class in college, but had not taken any courses in mathematical proof, much less Real Analysis. By the end of my first week of class I realized I was ill-prepared for the program.

The economics department held a wine and cheese reception at the end of the week, to welcome first-year graduate students. There I learned we had forty-three people in our class, including only five women. I also learned that most of the first year students, perhaps two thirds of the class, had received a full fellowship, which included the cost of tuition plus a stipend to cover living expenses. The University of Indiana had offered me a similar package, but I chose Northwestern's offer of admittance with no financial aid because I wanted the opportunity to attend a top-ten program. I took out a loan from the Federal Student Loan program to cover tuition—only $6,000 then—and my father lent me $500 a month to cover living expenses.

I had naively expected graduate school would be less structured than college, with seminars rather than lectures and frequent one-on-one discussions with professors. But Dr. B's talk had disabused me of that notion. This program, which I had so unwittingly entered, was even more structured than high school. The highly competitive, virtually all-male culture made it worse. Together in the same classes for most of the day, we all seemed to be checking each other out, as if we were bulls during rutting season, sizing each other up for the inevitable fight for dominance.

I had enough confidence in my math skills to believe I could understand anything if I worked hard enough at it and I thought my course work at Northwestern would be no different. I had less confidence in how well I would hold up emotionally.

The heartbreak from my failed relationship with Christy, along with the feeling I was utterly alone in this strange place, became almost unbearable. I often fantasized about suicide, although I never seriously considered actually doing it.

Then a remarkable series of events occurred that ended my thoughts of suicide and began to gradually lift me out of my depression.

Maybe Somebody Up There Does Like Me

On Friday evening, at the end of the first week of classes, I attended a picnic for first-year graduate students in all the schools across the university. Northwestern provided food and drinks plus made available a volleyball court. Upon arriving I joined a circle of classmates from the economics program. I couldn't have felt more nerdy, standing with these guys, nursing our beers, and discussing the fine points of the supply-side theory of economics—which Reagan used to hammer Carter in the presidential debates. I needed to get away and hopefully meet someone from outside the economics department. So I slipped away from my buddies and ambled towards the volleyball court.

As I stood waiting for my turn to get into the game a guy came up to me and said, "Hey Ira. Remember me? I'm

Seth. You and my brother Clifford were friends in grade school and I used to hang out with you, too."

Immediately I recognized the brother of the best friend I ever had, long ago in third grade. I asked Seth what Clifford was up to and Seth told me with a shrug that Clifford had taken a different path than either of us. He went on to tell me that Clifford had gone to a small college in upstate New York known for its hippie culture. He added that Clifford was still there as a fifth-year senior.

Wow, I thought to myself. *That sounds almost exactly like the school my step-sister Elizabeth just started at as a freshman a couple of weeks ago.* I asked Seth if Clifford was, by any chance, attending Bard College. Seth answered yes. I stood there silent for a few moments, dumbstruck by the coincidence. He and I talked a while longer and then joined the volleyball game. After the game we agreed we would have to get together again and exchanged phone numbers. Then I walked off to get a beer.

Just a few minutes later, a very attractive woman wearing tight jeans and a T-shirt came up to me. She said "Hi, Ira. Do you remember me?"

"Umm," I replied, trying to fathom this gift from heaven.

"I'm Joy Ballerini," she said. "We went to Andrew Warde together."

The name sounded familiar, but I just couldn't place her. *Stall for time,* I thought. I urged myself to say something, anything, to keep the conversation going. *Don't let this girl walk away. Man, is she hot.*

I replied, "Oh yeah. Now I remember. We were in some

classes together, weren't we?" thinking as soon as the words came out of my mouth that I couldn't have possibly said anything more lame.

Fortunately, she kept trying. "Yes," she said, "We were in psychology class together. I used to wake you up when the teacher called on you."

Now I remembered her. *Holy shit!* I thought to myself. *She didn't look like this in high school. Wow. What a transformation!*

I said, "Oh yeah. We had a lot of laughs in that class. So what brings you out to Northwestern?"

Then we started talking about old times and how we had landed there … She'd come to attend Northwestern's School of Communications Speech and Language Pathology program. She told me about her passion for working with children with cognitive disabilities. She had wanted to be a speech therapist since the age of thirteen, when she began babysitting for a child with severe developmental disabilities.

Before the evening ended I found Seth and introduced him to Joy. We agreed to go out to dinner and a comedy club the following weekend along with Mary, a new friend of Joy's. Joy and I also agreed to get together again within the next week or two to play raquetball.

I walked back to my room, elated I had just made two friends who were *not* in the economics program. The next morning I checked my mail and found a letter from Elizabeth. I couldn't believe my eyes when I read she had met this guy named Clifford who told her he used to be friends with me when we were kids. Then I noticed a small piece of paper folded into Elizabeth's letter. I unfolded the paper and discovered to my amazement that Clifford had written a note to me, which he had evidently asked Elizabeth to insert in her letter. The note read:

"Ira.
You're alive!
Let's meet again.
Clifford."

I will never know why Clifford chose the words, "You're alive," but his words shook me to my core. I knew then that the simple fact of my existence made a difference in the world. I would somehow make it work at Northwestern.

Hunkering Down

Having survived my meaning-of-life crisis, I settled into a routine that included studying, running, sleeping, and more studying. Following Dr. B's advice, I joined a study group that gradually expanded from one other person—a guy who had also gone to Fordham and had befriended me after learning that we had both been accepted to Northwestern—to several, as we and the rest of our classmates got to know each other. Classes and study group meetings alone took close to forty hours a week. I spent another twenty to thirty hours a week studying on my own.

It took a few weeks to understand that the first-year program was all about learning the basics of mathematical economics, the language economists use to speak to each other in peer reviewed journal articles. At this stage in our development, intellectual curiosity was a liability. Our professors expected nothing more—or less—of us than to absorb the nuggets of wisdom they imparted to us each day. Our opinions and ideas would not become relevant until we demonstrated mastery of the subject matter by passing the Prelim exam.

This expectation became abundantly clear to me one day when I visited my Macro Economics professor, Dr. W. A strong proponent of the Rational Expectations theory in vogue among conservative economists at the time, he made it the focus of his course. To my mind, the underlying premise of Rational Expectations, that people act rationally using the information they have at their disposal to maximize their self-interests, did not jibe with reality. I asked Dr. W whether and how Rational Expectations theory accounts for people who act irrationally, based on their emotions. At Fordham, my professors had encouraged this type of questioning. But Dr. W became visibly angry. He made a pretense of answering my question, but his manner and body language sent a clear message: "Don't waste my time asking irreverent and irrelevant questions. Your job as a first-year student is to learn what I teach, not to question it."

I realized then I had enrolled in something akin to special-forces boot camp for geeks. The program accepted a cadre of promising recruits and taught us the basic skills we needed to survive before winnowing our number to an elite squad of PhD candidates who demonstrated the intellectual fitness to move on to more advanced training. I knew now to ignore my intellectual curiosity and instead hunker down and focus my energy on the job at hand.

A Not So Foreign Land

Under the intense pressure of this boot camp, we jelled as a group. A core collection of perhaps twenty-five of us attended class together, studied together, ate lunch together, and went to the same dive bar in downtown Evanston together. The more time we spent together, the more insular we became. Many of us, myself included, developed a superiority complex; we enjoyed nothing more than to put down the MBA students we saw preening around campus in their suits and ties on their way to mock interviews.

Several of us, eager to demonstrate that our talents extended beyond using our well-honed math skills, ventured onto the field of athletics and formed an intramural softball team. Our team did about as well as one would expect from a group of economics geeks. Our opponents, mostly undergraduate frat jocks, clobbered us in every game. Our lone "moral victory" was not getting mercied the last game of the season.

As planned when we all met during the first-year picnic, Joy, her friend Mary, Seth, and I went out together the following Saturday night to dinner and a comedy club. The comedian was awful, but we made up for it by having lots of good laughs over dinner. Joy and I seemed to hit it off well. I could tell she had a great sense of humor because she laughed at all my jokes. I was not ready to get into a new romantic relationship, as I had not yet gotten over my break-up with Christy, but I liked Joy and wanted to see her again. Fortunately, she felt the same and accepted my invitation to play raquetball the following Saturday.

Much to my later embarrassment, Joy noticed me

checking out her legs during our first raquetball game—and I thought I had been discreet! I confirmed she did indeed have great legs and she, for some reason that still escapes me, agreed to play raquetball again the following Saturday.

Still just friends, we made Saturday morning raquetball a regular part of our week. Some time in late October or early November we added a weekly lunch date in the student union cafeteria to our routine. The first couple of times we met there I could feel my classmates watching our every step. I basked in their envy.

Over the next several weeks we found more things to do together—a free movie on campus, a trip to Chicago—and gradually grew closer. But despite our mutual physical attraction, the relationship remained purely platonic. We had become like the Bruce Willis and Cybil Sheppard characters in *Moonlighting*. "When will they ever get together?" our friends must have wondered.

Thanksgiving

If I could point to a moment when I began to feel at home in Evanston, it would be Thanksgiving dinner. Chris, widely considered one of the top students in the class and someone who shared my interest in philosophy, hosted the dinner. He invited all the first-year economics students he knew who stayed in Evanston for the long weekend, plus their significant others. About fifteen people attended; Joy went as my date. Two other women came with guys in the program.

Although happy to be invited, I was a little apprehensive about the dinner. I had never felt entirely comfortable in social gatherings with more than a few people unless I knew them all well. And despite all the time I spent with the other guys in the economics department—attending classes, eating lunch in the student union cafeteria and studying together—I still considered them to be no more than friendly acquaintances. I rarely socialized with any of them. A few of us occasionally went to the Orrington Hotel bar, the local dive in the center of Evanston, after our last class on Friday afternoon, but that was it. I felt lucky to have Joy in my life.

Chris' apartment, or more accurately, his two-bedroom house, was a cut above the student slum dwellings that most of us inhabited. Had it not been for the garage sale furniture and the eclectic mix of posters that decorated the walls, his place could easily have been mistaken for the home of a young professional couple. The large living room/dining room and full kitchen made it perfect for hosting a dinner for fifteen people.

Chris provided the turkey, the stuffing, and a few other essentials and we each brought a side dish, dessert, and/ or bottle of wine. Not having a clue how to cook something that anyone else would actually want to eat, I felt a weight come off my shoulders when Joy offered to bring a vegetable dish. Our feast included everything one would hope to see at a traditional Thanksgiving dinner: yams, baked potatoes, home-made cranberry sauce, bread, two vegetable dishes and, of course, apple and pumpkin pie for dessert. Even the dinners my mother served for Thanksgiving and Passover did not surpass the meal set before us.

Perhaps it was the aroma of the bread warming in the oven, along with the sight of the huge, perfectly golden-brown, seething-with-juices turkey that Chris brought to the table. Or maybe we just needed to have Joy and the other two women there to keep us from talking about economics. But something special happened during that dinner. All of us a long way from wherever we called home, we made each other our family for those few hours. We talked and laughed together as if we had known each other since childhood. I felt a sense of kinship and belonging I hadn't experienced since college graduation.

The party started at about 2 p.m. and was still going strong late into the evening. Only three or four people had left when, at midnight, we braved the cold and went to a park across the street to play touch football. When we returned, Chris served the most delicious turkey soup I had ever eaten—he'd started slow-cooking the remains of the turkey just after we finished the main meal. The party finally broke up not long after we ate the soup.

I wonder if the others at the party remember it so vividly. I think Joy's presence elevated the event from a really good Thanksgiving dinner to a magical evening. Joy and I, although more than just good friends by then, had not yet crossed the line to become romantic partners. Back then—in 1980—the term "friends with benefits" had not yet been invented. Even if it had, Joy would never have gone for it. Raised in a conservative family, she learned traditional values. A woman never asked the man for a date and never made the first move. She waited for the man to do so—that is, assuming she liked him enough to wait.

After we had finished eating, Joy and I sat on a couch next to each other. I put my arm around her shoulders. This was the first time I had touched her. Then, during the football game, I gently tackled her a few times. It would be another three months before we kissed for the first time. Joy had waited for me to make the first move. She must have liked me. We left Chris' house braced by the cold, the warmth of the soup in our bellies, the friendship we shared with the others at the party, and the affection we felt toward each other.

· · · · · · · · ·

Our relationship having progressed to a gray zone somewhere between platonic and romantic, Joy and I drove back to Connecticut in her car at Christmas break. During this trip Joy revealed a quality I had not seen in her before: quiet determination. Joy had told me she wanted to complete the fifteen-plus hour drive in one day. She arrived at my dorm the day of the trip at the appointed time of 6 a.m. with a cooler in the back seat containing all the food we would need to sustain us for the journey. We drove to Connecticut in record time, stopping only for carefully coordinated refueling/bathroom breaks along the way.

I clearly remember the precise moment I fell in love with her. A month after returning to Northwestern from Christmas break, I started feeling overwhelming fatigue. I tried to fight through it, but after three days of sleeping twelve hours and waking up exhausted I decided to follow Joy's advice and go to the infirmary. There I learned I had strep throat and pneumonia. I asked the doctor if he had any medicine for me take back to my dorm and he told me I wasn't going anywhere. I would be staying in the infirmary for the next several days.

I woke up the next day to find Joy in my room. She looked radiant in the kelly-green pants and yellow sweater she wore that day. Her energy and smile immediately lifted me out of the funk fatigue had caused. The concern I saw in her eyes when I met her gaze told me she cared deeply for me. At that moment I knew she was *the one*.

Shortly after my release from the infirmary Joy invited me to her place for a dinner of homemade stuffed shells. After we finished eating we sat down on a couch next to each other. I could feel the tension as we struggled to make conversation. Then I leaned over and kissed her for the first time.

Jim, Don, and the Toledo Marathon

By the time Joy and I played racquetball for the first time, my roommate Jim and I had already become fast friends. Jim's relaxed, easy-going persona stood in stark contrast to my initial impressions of my economics program classmates. And like me, he loved to talk. Having covered our life stories and reasons for being at Northwestern within the first few days of meeting each other, we moved on to general topics of interest, like the presidential race between Ronald Reagan and Jimmy Carter, the Ku Klux Klan rallies and counter rallies taking place in nearby Skokie, the proper role of government in a capitalist economy, and so on. Both of us interested in exploring new topics and ideas, we rarely ran out of things to talk about. My conversations with Jim became a welcome respite from the world of mathematical proofs and equations I inhabited for most of my days.

Jim, the quintessential extrovert, made friends easily. He also had a knack for bringing his friends from different walks of life together. A few days after we met, Jim invited me to go for pizza and beer with him and his new-found friends from his Organizational Behavior program. I joined them several more times that fall and by the end of our first trimester at Northwestern had gotten to know of few of them fairly well.

I learned during our frequent runs together that Jim's calm exterior belied an intense competitiveness that matched my own. We usually started out slowly enough to easily carry on a conversation, and then, after two or three miles, picked up the pace. We chased down anyone we saw in front of us running at a decent pace; we "dominated" countless runners who had no idea they were competing with us. A stronger runner than Jim, I usually pulled away from him when we got to within a mile or two of the finish. But just as often I held back, encouraging Jim to stay with me until I pulled away near the very end. Jim let me know he had added to his life goals beating me in a race some day.

Around mid-October, Jim and I started doing long runs on Sundays, increasing our distance by a mile or two each week until we reached eighteen miles the Sunday before Christmas break. This naturally led to talk about running a marathon—Jim had run the 1979 NYC Marathon, the year I dropped out. Jim apparently also had talked up the idea of a marathon with Don, one of his friends who by then had also become a good friend of mine. Always up for an adventure, Don agreed to give it a try. Upon returning from Christmas break, the three of us began training together.

When Jim and Don got Lance, another friend of theirs—with a car—interested, I knew the marathon talk had become serious. Jim and Don assigned themselves the task of finding a suitable venue. They both got a kick out of finding quirky, out-of-the-way places—the towns and cities most people ignore when they travel long distances on the Interstate. They especially liked to find postcards—the tackier, the better—from these places. They searched for a spring marathon in a location within reasonable driving distance of Evanston that fit this criterion. Familiar with Toledo mainly as the home of Klinger, the cross-dressing orderly in *M.A.S.H.*, they settled on the Toledo Heart-Watchers Marathon. I agreed, but for different reasons. I wanted to run a sub-three-hour marathon and knew my best chance would be on a flat course with few enough runners to enable me to run unimpeded at the beginning of the race. The Toledo Heart-Watchers Marathon perfectly met these criteria. The fact that Lance had a friend near Toledo who said he would put us up the night before the race sealed the deal. Now, with everything else in place, all we had to do was train for the race.

Finally, the day of our big adventure arrived, in April 1981. The four of us, plus another of Lance's friends who came along to take pictures and cheer us on, piled into the car. Joy sent us off, giving us sandwiches to eat along the way. We left about an hour behind schedule, consuming the sandwiches within a half hour of leaving Evanston.

Destination: University of Toledo. There we would register for the race and do our carbo-loading with a spaghetti dinner. We stopped along the way to look for postcards, putting us further behind schedule and then, as we approached the University of Toledo, made several wrong turns. By the time we arrived at the registration site, dinner had ended. Only the race organizers and a few runners remained. Not having eaten since we devoured Joy's sandwiches a few hours earlier, we were ravenous. Fortunately, the race organizers allowed us to register. They also found a couple of uneaten trays of spaghetti for us. We thanked them profusely and greedily wolfed down our dinner.

By the time we finished eating, it was close to nine. I was anxious to get going. We might have done that had Jim and Don not discovered some pinball machines on the way out. A half hour of playing pinball later, we finally set out for Lance's friend's house.

After about forty-five minutes of driving Lance announced we were lost. Afraid I would not get the sleep I needed to achieve my sub-three-hour marathon goal, I felt my pulse quicken and my neck and shoulders stiffen with tension. For everyone else, getting lost was part of the adventure, but I became entirely focused on the race. It was like the bus rides to the cross country meets in high school all over again, except this time I was accepted, even with my over-the-top intensity. We finally arrived at the house at about eleven. It was a good thirty-minute drive from the race starting area and the race was scheduled to start at 8:30, so we would have to get up by seven. By then, I didn't want to talk to anyone; I just wanted to go to bed. Seeing how wound up I was, the rest of the guys let me have the only available bedroom while they all slept on the floor in the living room.

I awoke the next morning fully rested and pumped for the race. We ate a quick breakfast, thanked Lance's friend for his hospitality, and headed back to the University of

Toledo, where the race would start and end. On our way there we talked mainly about the weather: 38 degrees, strong winds and rain. I told Jim, Don, and Lance that these conditions actually were not bad at all for running a marathon, but I don't think I convinced anyone.

We made it to the starting area without incident and I got out of car feeling like a bundle of energy. After checking in, I jogged for a few minutes and then did some wind sprints to loosen up, while most of the rest of the crowd stood by, huddling against the cold. I waited until the last possible minute and then stripped down to my singlet and shorts. By then the rain had turned into sleet. I was freezing, but I knew I would warm up within a few minutes.

The course was straight out with no turns for exactly 13.1 miles and then straight back along the same route. I planned to run the first half of the race at an easy pace and then run the second half as hard as I could. Jim adopted the same strategy and we started out running together. Facing a twenty-plus-mile-an-hour headwind, I expected our pace to be slow, but we pounded out one 6:45 mile after another. (A three hour marathon translates to a 6:43 pace.) Still feeling as energetic as I did at the start, I picked up the pace and left Jim behind just after passing the twelve-mile marker. I reached the halfway point in exactly one and a half hours.

When I turned around and began running with the wind at my back I felt a rush of energy unlike anything I had ever experienced before—or since—in a race. I ran hard the entire way back, gradually increasing my pace as I got closer to the finish line. For the last ten miles or so

I felt a thud of pain in my thighs each time my feet hit
the ground. But that only made me want to run harder.
And still feeling boundless energy, I could. I finished in
2:54:32—twenty-fifth of 400 runners. I covered the second half of the race at slightly better than a 6:30 per mile
pace—better than I thought I could run in my wildest
imagination.

Looking back, the last ten miles of that race is a good
metaphor for the next thirty years or so of my life after
high school. I still felt pain from the hits I took during
my childhood, but instead of letting it slow me down, I
used it as a motivator to push myself harder. Beginning
in college and throughout my career I demonstrated to
myself over and over again I had overcome my mother's
verbal abuse, my father's inattention, and bullying from
classmates. At each step along my career I strived to be
better than all my peers, to prove I deserved to move
up to the next level. Not until I learned to accept my
parents for who they were, even with all their flaws, and
accept my own limitations was I was able to stop pushing myself so hard.

. . . .

My first couple of weeks at Northwestern had become
a distant memory by the time I ran the Toledo Marathon.
What had once seemed so alien—the flatness of the terrain, the tiny apartment I shared with Jim, even the language of mathematical economics—had become familiar.
I had long since gotten to know most of my classmates
and had become friends with several of them. My chance
meeting with Joy had evolved into a serious relation-

ship. And I considered Jim and Don to be close friends. Evanston, as much as any place I had lived before, had become my home. But by spring time, decisions had to be made.

CHAPTER 13
DECISIONS, DECISIONS

Castles in the Sky

I believe the countless small decisions we make every day, more than luck or the big decisions that seem important at the time, shape the person we become. But every so often we come to a fork in the road where the choice we make has a profound impact for the rest of our lives. As the end of the academic year approached, I faced two such decisions. I spent weeks wrestling with the first. The second was obvious. In both cases I made the right choice.

I approached the more difficult decision, whether I should stay in the economics PhD program, in the same analytical manner I had used in the past to make important decisions. I developed a list of pluses and minuses. I came up with a Plan B and when that didn't work out, I came up with a plan C. I talked it over numerous times with Joy, Jim, and my friends from the economics program. And after all this I made what my gut told me was the right decision.

The other decision, whether I should stay in Evanston if I did drop out of the economics program, required very little contemplation. I knew my only real choice was to stay. Joy had another full year to go to complete her program and I wanted to stay in Evanston to be with her. After our first kiss in February there was no turning back. Our relationship quickly grew from just good friends with the possibility of something more to a deep love for each other built on a foundation of friendship. I didn't have a Plan B for this decision and I didn't need one. Don, Jim, and I had talked about rooming together off-campus. When Jim found a three bedroom apartment, I readily signed on.

Two main concerns drove my thinking about staying in the economics program. First, I wondered whether a career in economics would be intellectually stimulating. Economics as a discipline was at a low point at the time. People both within and outside the profession questioned whether economics deserved to be called a science. Unlike the hard sciences, economic theory did not rely on repeatable testing of hypotheses of how things work in the real world. Instead it relied on mathematical models based on questionable assumptions, like the premise that people always act in a rational manner.

The better I understood the models I had learned in my macroeconomics class that spring, the more skeptical I became. These models started with broad assumptions about the economy and ended with outcomes that suggested a preferred economic policy. I noticed the outcomes of these models usually coincided with the political slant of the university where their authors were employed. I began to wonder whether the authors of some of these models hadn't chosen their desired outcome first and then identified the assumptions that would cause the model to go there.

My microeconomics class consisted mainly of highly abstract mathematical proofs of theorems regarding how individuals behave in a market economy. The proofs relied on not only calculus, but also on more advanced branches of math like real analysis and topology. I could understand the proofs, but only after spending several hours after each class going through each one step by step.

Practitioners of this brand of economics, I observed, placed a high value on the elegance of a proof, almost as much as on the proof's economic meaningfulness. Like beauty in the physical world, elegance in a mathematical proof is difficult to define. No one definition exists that everyone agrees to. I understood it to mean a simple, straightforward, yet innovative solution to a problem. This class taught me to recognize and appreciate elegance in a mathematical proof.

Near the end of the trimester our professor introduced us to *Theory of Value: An Axiomatic Analysis of Economic Equilibrium*. This book, as unintelligible to the non-mathematician as its title suggests, is widely considered to be one of the most important works in mathematical economics. Using a novel approach, it proved that perfect competition is the most efficient economic system. Its author, Gerard Debreu, was awarded a Nobel Prize for the work he did leading up to this book.

We covered only the first chapter of the book in class. But beguiled by the elegance of the proofs in this book, I found it impossible to put down. For about a week I did little else as I plowed my way through, page by page. I probably understood only about half of what I read, but that was enough for me to appreciate the significance of Debreu's achievement.

But along with my appreciation came a realization that

this book was based entirely on deductive reasoning. It bore no relation to what I observed in the real world. I began to see it as a beautiful, delicate, intricately constructed castle in the sky held together by flimsy assumptions—a small change in any one of the assumptions and the whole house could come crashing down. I had been seduced by the elegance of Debreu's proofs, but ultimately found it to be unsatisfactory. I needed to be more grounded in reality.

Joy helped to pull me down to earth. We studied together at the library on Friday nights and after leaving walked along the lake shore to the house where she rented a room. During these walks, I talked to Joy about the angst I was feeling about a career in economics. She did exactly what I needed most—she listened. She took the time to understand my conflicting feelings of fascination and disillusionment with economics. She understood the battle raging inside me between not wanting to quit and needing to do something that mattered in the real world. And by her listening and understanding, she let me know without having to say it out loud that she would be there for me, no matter what I chose to do.

. . . .

I began to focus on a related concern—how I would support myself if I stayed in the program. Although not a star, I had overcome my early doubts about whether I could keep up with the work and had done reasonably well. I think I ranked somewhere near the fiftieth percentile of students in the program. Normally that would have been good enough to be assured financial support. But we had been told that with the Reagan cuts to the National

Science Foundation—a major source of funding for the school—there would be less money to go around.

More important than the money itself was the message that came with it. Northwestern based its financial decisions entirely on merit. We all understood that a decision by a school in any field not to provide financial support to a PhD candidate after his first year carried with it the stigma that the school was unwilling to invest in his future. As a result, most people who did not receive financial support dropped out of the program. If they wanted to continue to pursue a PhD they transferred to a lower-ranked school. While I waited to get an answer from Northwestern about the financial support they would provide, I received an unsolicited full fellowship offer from Fordham to enter its PhD program. I didn't consider this offer because Fordham was not an elite school and did not have a top-ten economics program.

Anticipating I might not make the cut at Northwestern, I decided to hedge my bet. I knew an advanced degree would significantly enhance my value in the job market so I resolved not to leave the program without first earning my Master's degree. Typically, PhD students at Northwestern earned their Master degrees by passing the Prelim Exam. This test was notoriously difficult; fewer than half the people in any one sitting passed. Many of the people who passed did so on their second or third try.

Fortunately Northwestern offered a second path to earning a Master's degree. Students with a 3.0 or better grade point average could earn a degree by writing a Master's thesis and successfully defending it in front of a panel of professors. During my senior year at Fordham I had written an honors thesis on the influence of classical economists such as Adam Smith and David Ricardo on Karl Marx's seminal work, *Das Kapital*. I pulled this thesis from the box of papers I had written at Fordham, put a new cover on it and presented it as my Master's thesis.

I did this with a clear conscience. I had done all the work to produce the thesis, just not at Northwestern. I knew the graduate student affairs chairman, Dr B, was well aware of the fact that I hadn't worked on my thesis with anyone at Northwestern. I also knew he had only to look at my application to see that I had written the paper while at Fordham. He scheduled my defense without questioning where or when I wrote the thesis.

At my defense I faced a panel of three professors. They gave me fifteen minutes to present an overview of my thesis and then began firing questions at me. Not expecting this fusillade, I nearly panicked. I became acutely aware of the sweat trickling from my armpits down the sides of my body. But I managed to keep my cool. I gave credible, if not insightful, answers to most of their questions. Mercifully, the inquisition ended after about 45 minutes. Dr. B gave no indication of whether I passed or failed. He just told me he would be getting back to me soon.

About a week later, after classes had ended, I received a letter from Dr. B informing me I had passed the defense and therefore had earned my Master's degree. The letter went on to say the school had granted me a full tuition scholarship to return for my second year in the program and I should expect to work ten to fifteen hours a week as a teaching assistant. The letter concluded by saying the offer was contingent on passing the Prelim Exam in the fall. I assumed, perhaps incorrectly, I would not be paid for my teaching assistant duties and planned accordingly.

I had already made up my mind, but didn't realize it at the time. Instead of focusing on Plan A, which would have meant preparing for the Prelim Exam, I concentrated my efforts on finding a job. I started with the idea of getting one that would allow me to work full-time during the summer and then scale back to about ten hours a week so I could stay in school and make enough money to cover living expenses—I needed only about $450 a month, as my share of the rent for the apartment Jim found was only $125. First, I checked to see whether any professors in the economics department needed a research assistant. None of them did. Next I tried the Finance Department in the business school. Again, no luck. I scoured the whole campus and found nothing.

Finally, I did the unthinkable. I went in to the MBA program Career Placement Office to see if they could help. The office manager there told me what I already knew: the MBA career placement program was intended just for MBA students. On a whim I asked her if I could use the resources in the library. Much to my surprise, she said yes. That marked the beginning of the end of my career in academia.

The next day I went back to the MBA Career Placement Office and started looking through the shelves hoping I might find something useful. I saw books on resume writing, how to interview for a job, how to dress for success, and the like. I also saw binder after binder filled with annual reports, 10k reports, news clippings, and other information about companies that recruited MBAs at

Northwestern. Then I found what I was looking for: a binder filled with letters from local companies notifying the Office of positions they were trying to fill. I found several positions that intrigued me. But the position that interested me most was Research Associate for a small unit within the Blue Cross Blue Shield Association that did strategy consulting. They were looking for someone with exceptional quantitative skills as well as the ability to see the big picture—no experience required. It seemed like a perfect fit.

A few days later I received a letter inviting me to come in for interviews. It would be a long day. I was to arrive at nine and then meet with five individuals plus two of the same people over lunch. I found myself for the first time since I was a five-year-old thanking my mother for the lessons in table manners. I showed up for my interviews wearing the only suit I owned—a brown tweed. Had I realized how inappropriately I was dressed, I might have been more nervous. But I felt completely at ease. With each interview I became more interested in the job. I could tell from the body language of my future colleagues the feeling was mutual. At the end of the day, Paul, the Executive Director of the department, invited me into his office for a short chat before I left. There he offered me the Research Associate position at an annual salary of $22,800. I thought he had made a mistake. I couldn't believe how much he had just offered me. It was more than four times as much as I needed to live on! Stunned, I didn't know what to say. Paul told me to think it over for a few days and then get back to him. A couple of days later I received a formal offer letter. By then I had already decided to take the job. With that, my career as an academic ended.

· · · · · · · · ·

With this job offer, I knew I would stay in Evanston with Joy. But still, I held back in our relationship out of fear we might become too close. I didn't want to get hurt again and didn't want to hurt Joy. I enjoyed the time we spent together and I knew my feelings toward her had progressed far beyond fondness, but I somehow felt safer keeping her at a distance. What if we did become closer, I worried. What if we fell in love, got married, and then discovered we were not right for each other? I didn't want to repeat the mistake my parents had made.

I remembered the warning my father had given me four years earlier about Kathy. She had been my first and only girlfriend for three years when my father spoke to me. He expressed his concern I was headed down a slippery slope that would eventually lead to marriage. He told me he liked Kathy well enough, but thought she lacked intellectual curiosity. Aware that she hoped to one day teach at the same parochial school she had attended as a child, he feared I might find myself trapped in a marriage where I would be expected to follow the same Catholic doctrine that had oppressed Jews for centuries. My father urged me to see other women before it was too late.

I reacted angrily to the advice. I told him Kathy and I had never talked about marriage and the notion we would unknowingly go down that path was insulting. Then I accused him of being a hypocrite and a bigot. But four years later, his advice gave me pause. Since I had rejected the notion of a caring God, any woman with an unquestioning belief in the dogma of her religion would have been a terrible match for me.

I had to admit Joy and Kathy had a lot in common. Joy grew up less than a mile from Kathy and had attended the same parochial school and high school. Both got straight As before going to a Connecticut state school on a full academic scholarship. And if that were not enough, both looked forward to a career working with children. Both were the youngest in their families and had doting mothers.

A final commonality: both lived less than an hour and a half from New York City, but rarely visited as children because their parents were afraid that, with all the black people roaming the city, they might get mugged.

The similarities between Joy and Kathy, incredible as they were, ended there. Joy decided to leave the comforts and safety of home for Northwestern. She loved her family but needed to live apart from them. She went to Northwestern not only because it had the top-ranked Speech Pathology program in the country, but also because, 800 miles from Fairfield, it gave her the opportunity to escape the confines of home and begin her life as an independent adult. Years later Joy told me she could feel a weight lift from her shoulders as she drove by herself from Connecticut to Evanston that September. After college, Kathy went to work at her parochial school.

The following August, Joy graduated from her speech therapy program and took a job in a school district not far from Evanston. A month later we moved into an apartment together. And so began the next phase of our lives.

. . . .

I had Joy in my life—pun intended. But I almost blew it. I waited for almost two years to pop the question while Joy and I shared an apartment, a bed, and a life with each other. We had a great life together.

But how could I know it would remain that way? What if Joy turned into my mother: fat, insecure, and bitter? What if Joy discovered the real me, the guy who everyone liked to pick on in school, and stopped loving me? I knew these fears were baseless and we lived in an uncertain world, where nothing is guaranteed. I needed to take a leap of faith that our love would last. I finally took the leap, and landed on the other side. My love for Joy overcame my fears. She, instead of my hateful, bitter, narcissistic, always-screaming-at-me-for-something mother became the primary female influence in my life.

In retrospect, my doubts about getting married had little to do with Joy. They were about my fear of following in my father's footsteps, chained to a woman he no longer found attractive and with whom he no longer had any common interests. And worst of all, someone he argued with every time he saw her. I worried that Joy would become my mother.

How could I have been so wrong, I think now as I look back over thirty-three years of a happy marriage. Joy was and still is everything my mother was not.

CHAPTER 14
WIFE OF THE CENTURY

Joy and I married in 1984. We moved from Chicago to Minneapolis, Dallas, New York, Stamford, Amherst, and finally to Ann Arbor—six moves within sixteen years, all but once for me to advance my career. For Joy this meant resigning from her job, saying goodbye to her friends, and starting all over.

We have had a great marriage, but it was not always easy.

Initial Impressions

Joy was pretty when I met her at Northwestern—long, thin legs, dark brown hair that flowed to her shoulders, and brown eyes that melted me whenever I looked into them.

Quiet, soft-spoken, and painfully shy, Joy rarely expressed an opinion and hardly ever spoke out when in a group of more than the two of us. She would tell me after getting together with my friends from the economics department that they intimidated her. She couldn't keep up with us, she admitted, sometimes with tears in her eyes, as we competed to make the most clever argument for why it is possible to fit an infinite number of angels on the head of a pin. Joy's lack of self-confidence belied an intelligence that enabled her to get straight As at every school she attended, including Northwestern, rated the top school in the country in her field.

I knew the smartest person in the room at these gatherings had nothing on her. Joy was brilliant, but in a different way than me and my preening friends. She had—and more than thirty-five years later still has—a genius for identifying on the spot simple but effective interventions that make a world of difference to her clients.

Joy also had a great sense of humor. How could she not when she laughed at all of my jokes? Joy could be funny herself, too. At the beginning her jokes reflected a sweet, innocent persona. We once stayed overnight at a campground and the next morning saw a sign that said "Lots for Sale." I asked rhetorically how much the lots might cost. Joy replied, "A lot." Over the years she has become a little less innocent and her jokes more biting. We often laugh about how the sweet thing I married has turned into a female version of me.

A Peripatetic Life Once More

Our first move, from Chicago to Minneapolis, was the most difficult for Joy. I had accepted a position in the management consulting division of Touche Ross, then one of the Big Eight accounting firms. I saw this move as a great career opportunity. Experience at Touche Ross would add cache to my resume and Minneapolis was a hot-bed of managed care activity, a new industry in which I wanted to focus my career.

I moved to Minneapolis about six weeks before Joy. Working sixty to seventy hours per week, I quickly became immersed in my new job. Joy, meanwhile, packed our belongings, arranged to turn our utilities off in Evanston and on in Minneapolis, and did whatever else was necessary to prepare for the move. She also updated her resume and started making contacts with potential employers.

We hit the home stretch on a project I had been working on the day Joy arrived. For the next three weeks, my sixty to seventy hours per week turned into eighty to ninety. Joy and I barely saw each other. For all practical purposes, Joy had moved by herself into an apartment full of boxes in a place she had never been to before. When the project ended I came home to an apartment bereft of boxes and everything in its proper place. She told me she had lined up several interviews for herself.

Neither of us realized we could have expected it then, but our move to Minneapolis was just a warm-up to a series of events that would severely test the strength of our marriage and each of us individually.

Two's a Marriage, Four's a Family

When we were in our twenties, Joy wanted more than anything else to have children. I did too, but I did not think I was ready.

We were living in Dallas and had been trying for a pregnancy for about a year when a home test revealed Joy was pregnant for the first time. The timing could not have been better. We had long since planned a trip to go hiking in Big Bend, which meant we would have plenty of time to talk about the baby's name, how we would furnish his or her room, what we would do about our child's religious upbringing, and so forth. We quickly decided on a boy's name, Alan David, in honor of our fathers. We couldn't agree on a girl's name, but this debate only heightened our excitement—we would soon be the parents of a real live baby!

The day after our return, Joy scheduled a visit with her obstetrician, Dr. S, who we privately called Dr. Koppel due to his uncanny resemblance to the late-night news anchor Ted Koppel. But this routine visit never happened. Two or three days after our return, Joy woke up at about two in the morning bleeding heavily. She woke me up a half hour later when the pain started. Still groggy from a deep sleep, I mumbled to Joy that everything would be okay. But by then her pain had become almost unbearable. Joy knew everything was not okay. In a much louder, more strident voice, Joy told me to get out of bed, call Dr. Koppel's answering service and start getting dressed, in that order. I called and a few minutes later Dr. Koppel called back. He told us to go immediately to the emergency room, where he would meet us in twenty minutes. There we learned that Joy had indeed been pregnant and had just suffered a miscarriage. Upset by the loss myself, I didn't fully appreciate until years afterwards just how painful the experience had been for Joy, both physically and emotionally.

The second pregnancy happened when I was in Fort Wayne, Indiana, on a round of interviews for a job at Lincoln National. We had arranged for Joy to fly to Fort Wayne that afternoon so she and I could have dinner with my potential new boss and his wife. The following day Joy and I were to take a tour of the Fort Wayne environs with a realtor the company had found for us. Early that afternoon, shortly before her scheduled departure time, Joy called to tell me she was beginning to experience the same bleeding and pain she'd had leading up to her miscarriage several months earlier. I should have ended the interviews right then and caught the first plane back home, but instead I let reason and logic overwhelm my emotions. Concerned I might lose the job opportunity if I left, I asked Joy if she needed me at home. She agreed I should finish the visit as planned. Later that night Joy miscarried again, this time eight weeks into her pregnancy. The guilt I felt the next morning as I talked to her on the phone while she lay alone in her hospital room still haunts me.

The day had started out perfectly the third time. That morning, to celebrate my thirty-third birthday, Joy took me to Sunday brunch at The Mansion, widely considered one of the best restaurants in Dallas. After a meal that surpassed our expectations, she took me to Plano to visit the Legacy Book store, one of the largest independent book stores in the country. There Joy gave me the best possible birthday gift: as much time as I wanted to wander around the store before selecting a few books to take home. I planned to cap off the day by going for a long run in the sunny sixty-degree weather.

We got home and I relaxed for a few minutes with *The New York Times* in the family room while Joy straightened up in the kitchen. I shouted my running plans to Joy and made my way upstairs to get changed. But Joy asked me to stop. Her eyes moist, she told me she had been bleeding all day. She had kept it to herself for fear of ruining my day. But by now the bleeding had become heavy and the discomfort she felt earlier in the day had morphed into pain that was becoming more intense by the minute.

Almost without thinking, we numbly went through the now familiar routine of calling Dr. Koppel's answering service and heading to the emergency room. There, one of Dr. Koppel's colleagues confirmed that Joy had just suffered her third early-term miscarriage in less than a year. Our grief at this loss was far greater than the first two times—now we worried we would never have a child of our own. We decided the fourth time would be the last, regardless of the outcome.

About ten weeks into her fourth pregnancy Joy called me at work. I sat in stunned silence while she told me she was bleeding heavily. She needed me to come home right away to go with her to the obstetrician. During my hour-and-a-half commute from mid-town Manhattan to our house in North Stamford I tried to imagine a scenario that would result in a positive outcome, but I couldn't do it. I finally arrived home, expecting to find Joy curled up in a ball, sobbing. Instead, she projected an almost business-like demeanor. She had made an appointment with her doctor and we needed get going right away. I knew Joy wanted to be left alone in her thoughts, so we drove to the appointment in silence. Shortly after we arrived, an attendant called Joy's name and led us to an examination room. A few minutes later Dr. G—or Stephanie, as she preferred we call her—arrived. Joy and I maintained a calm visage that belied the almost unbearable tension we felt as Stephanie prepared Joy for a sonogram. Finally, after what seemed like hours but must have been less than a minute, Stephanie showed us the image on the sonogram. Joy burst out crying and I looked on in silent awe as Stephanie pointed out the beating heart of a healthy fetus.

Seven months later, with Joy now a full three weeks past her due date, Stephanie ordered her to the hospital for an induced delivery. After we arrived and got settled, the delivery room nurse hooked Joy up with two intravenous drips, one with Pitocin to induce dilation and the other with an epidural to staunch the pain. She also gave Joy a sedative to help her relax. I asked, only half joking, if I could have some of the sedative too.

After twenty-three hours, the initial thrill of our arrival had long since turned into boredom. I passed the time watching Joy sleep, checking the monitors and reading Michael Crichton's book, *Congo*. Finally, Stephanie entered the room to check on Joy. Upon completing her examination, she announced Joy had dilated enough to begin pushing the baby out and instructed the nurse to stop the epidural drip. Excited to put into practice our Lamaze training, I sat next to her, held her hand and began coaching her on her breathing. I had expected the delivery to take no more than twenty to thirty minutes. I could barely contain my excitement. But then, as twenty minutes turned into an hour, and an hour turned into first two hours and then three, my thoughts shifted from the baby to Joy. I watched in awe as she kept pushing, seemingly impervious to the pain. Not once during the entire three hours did she ask to stop or lash out at me or anyone else in the room. She exhibited strength and courage I hadn't realized she possessed. The only thing in my experience that remotely compared was running a marathon. But while I could usually find a nice comfortable pace, Joy was sprinting for a minute or more at a time, taking less and less time between sprints to rest as the day wore on.

Finally, we saw the baby crown. Stephanie told us he would emerge in just a few minutes. Squeamish about blood and wanting to remain conscious, I quickly moved to a position behind Joy. Then Stephanie held up a baby boy. I looked on in horror—our baby was blue! I started to panic. *Why is he not breathing? Why isn't Stephanie doing something?* But about three seconds later, before I had time to run out into the hall and scream "Emergency," Alan started wailing and turned a more normal pinkish color. A wave of relief washed over me. A moment later I felt an outpouring of love unlike anything I had ever felt before. Nothing else in the world mattered. My love for Alan had no beginning or end—it was infinite. All I needed was to know I had a son and he was healthy.

A couple of hours later I went home exhausted, overwhelmed by my love for Alan, and feeling a heightened respect for Joy that made me love her more than ever. I had never thought I could enjoy such happiness.

Our second son, Sam, joined us three years later. Raising the two boys was challenging at times but we also had lots of fun. They both are now well on their way to living happy, independent adulthoods. They have grown up wonderfully.

Wife—and Daughter-in-Law—of the Century

My mother, prone to hyperbole, said to Joy one day after she had done a favor for her, "You must be the wife of the century." Much to Joy's chagrin the label stuck. Over the years I have bought a nightgown and any number of T-shirts with the custom-inscribed words, "Wife of the Century" written boldly across the front.

I frequently addressed birthday and anniversary cards to Joy as W.O.T.C. Joy said she didn't want to be the wife of the century—too much pressure to keep up that standard. As the year 2000 approached, Joy said she was happy that somebody else would take over the mantle of Wife of the Century. I replied she was one of the early favorites for Wife of the Millennium.

Of course all this talk about Joy being the Wife of the Century was just a joke. But just beneath the surface has been real and ongoing dialogue about our relationship with each other. Joy is a truly amazing person. It is rare after a visit with old friends or family for no one to remind me how lucky I am to have her. I sometimes wonder how lucky they think she is to have me.

During Joy's many trips back to Fairfield when I did not accompany her she made a point to visit my mother.

Joy was not just the Wife of the Century, she was the Daughter-in-law of the Century.

CHAPTER 15
A RUNNING LIFE...OR NOT

Running had been an important part of my life since I started as a fourteen-year-old freshman in high school. Back then running was my escape from a dysfunctional home life and the taunts of bullies at school. Running gave me confidence. It was much more than something I did; it was an integral part of my self-identity. Twenty-five years later, when Joy, Sam, and I moved to Ann Arbor, I still thought of myself as a runner. Whenever someone asked me to "Tell me about yourself" during a networking interview, I included running as part of my answer. I had run several marathons, which I considered as important an accomplishment as anything I had done at work.

I ran the two best races of my life that year at Northwestern. I ran a 10k in 35.57, finishing in seventh place—out of about 300—after catching and sprinting by a guy I had been dueling with for the entire race. The second was the 1981 Toledo Heart-Watchers Marathon described earlier.

My next three marathons did not go so well. Each time I had severe insomnia the week before the race that prevented me from running nearly as fast as I knew I could. In 1983, two years after my Toledo exploits, I dropped out of the Chicago Marathon. Four years later I ran the Minneapolis Marathon, hell-bent on and in shape to break

2:50—the qualifying time to run the Boston Marathon. I slept no more than five hours each of the four nights before the race. Despite training harder than I ever had before, I struggled to finish in 3:07. Next came the 1998 Newport, Rhode Island, Ocean City Marathon.

Jim, Don, Lance, and I decided to go to Newport for a reunion and the marathon. Jim's, Don's and Lance's wives and Lance's two small children also came along. Joy stayed in Minneapolis, but Edythe, living in Providence at the time, also came to watch. Once again I had trained hard and expected to do well. That is, until the week before the race. This time was worse than the others, by far. I felt absolutely miserable. Jim and Don had to cajole me into joining them for dinner the night before. I hadn't seen either of them for three years but I just wanted to sleep. I managed to get six or seven hours of sleep that night but I felt worse the next morning, race day, than I had the day before. That morning I made a pact with myself. I decided I was going to finish no matter what. Having twice dropped out of a marathon, I had to prove to myself I could finish no matter how much it hurt.

The course, two loops around Newport, was beautiful, with spectacular views of the ocean and mansions built during the Gilded Age. I did not appreciate any of it because I was struggling from the beginning. By the time I completed the first loop I was trading off between running and walking. As I continued, the situation just got worse and worse until it got to the point where every step was a new experience in pain. I don't know how I did it, but after four hours I managed to finish the race, weaving from one side of the road to the other as I staggered across the finish line. Edythe told me later I was as white as a ghost, but

I did recover and was able to move around again in about an hour.

Finishing under those conditions was an incredibly stupid thing to do—I could have done serious harm to myself. If someone had asked me then why it was so important to finish, I would have just said I wanted to prove to myself I could do it. But I couldn't have told him why. Now, with the benefit of thirty years of perspective, I think I have an idea of why it was so important. It had become a kind of metaphor for life. Despite the fact that I had done exceedingly well in college, was off to a great start in my career and was married to a wonderful woman, I still had to prove over and over to myself I was worthy. And even though I had overcome some serious obstacles to get where I was, I still needed to prove to myself I could overcome whatever new obstacles came my way. So despite finishing in well over four hours, completing this marathon was a watershed event for me. It boosted my self-confidence at a time when I badly needed it. It would be fifteen years before I ran another marathon and I would never again try to finish just to prove I could.

· · · · · · · · ·

After staggering across the finish line at Ocean City, I vowed never to run a marathon again. And when I stopped running marathons, I stopped running in races altogether. I had lost my competitive fire, or more accurately, had redirected it toward work. I continued to run almost every day, but I rarely pushed myself very hard. Twelve years after Newport, I had gained close to twenty pounds.

Getting My Running Mojo Back

I hadn't realized just how far I had fallen out of shape until one unseasonably warm day in January of 2001 when we were living in Amherst. I got an urge to run home from the far end of the bike trail, so I arranged for Joy to drop me off there on our way back from doing errands. I hadn't run more than six miles at a time in the four years since we had moved to Amherst. But it was a beautiful day and I felt great.

I started out at slightly faster than my normal pace, letting my thoughts meander from topic to topic as I usually did during most of my long, slow runs. For me, running was a form of meditation. My mind would focus entirely on the present. I observed thoughts going by but I rarely stopped to follow up on one of them. At least a couple of times, though, my thoughts drifted to a difficult problem at work and before I realized I was thinking about the problem, I had solved it.

This time I noticed the seven mile marker on the side of the trail just minutes after I started my run. The marker having broken my reverie, I decided to take the opportunity to measure my pace. I had only a vague idea of how fast I usually ran, as I had never bothered to check out the distances of the routes; I guessed that I was running about seven minutes a mile. At the six-mile marker I looked at my watch; it said 9:05. *That can't be right*, I thought. *They must have misplaced the marker. My time will be much faster for the next mile.* I reset my watch and started running again, picking up the pace a little for good measure. When I reached the five-mile marker, I looked at my watch again. It said 8:35. I couldn't believe it. I used to run at about a 6:30 per mile pace on my faster runs. I decided to push hard this time to reassure myself I could still run fast if I wanted to. When I reached the four-mile marker at 7:45 I was crestfallen. The best I could do on a day I felt great was a 7:45 mile. Worse than that, I still had over four miles to go and I had already worn myself out. I slowed down to a comfortable jog, thinking I would take it easy the rest of the way. But fatigue took over. By the time I passed the two-mile marker my comfortable jog had turned into an all-out effort to reach my house without having to stop to walk. Finally I arrived at home, exhausted. My thighs and calves throbbed with pain as I limped up the driveway to my house. But the disappointment I leveled at myself felt far worse. I pledged then and there to lose weight and get back in shape.

Losing weight proved to be surprisingly easy for me—I just stopped eating fried foods, stopped drinking two to three large glasses of orange juice every morning, and started running more. As I lost weight, it became easier to run and as I ran longer and faster more weight came off—a virtuous circle.

By the summer of 2001 I had lost most of the twenty pounds and gotten myself back into running shape. Now on my fast runs I averaged about 7:00 a mile—not as fast as I used to run but not bad for a forty-three-year-old. That summer I ran a 10K race—my first race in years—and a five-mile race. I finished in the top ten in the five-mile race, averaging 6:40 a mile. I had my running mojo back.

Ann Arbor

In late 2001 we moved so I could take a position at MedStat, now a part of IBM, in Ann Arbor, managing relationships with clients who licensed our "analytically-ready" medical claims database and reporting systems. If that sounds like a mouthful, it is, because our systems were extremely complex. My clients were Blue Cross plans, HMOs, and the like. I loved my new job.

I started at MedStat a month before Joy and the boys moved to Ann Arbor. I missed them, but at least between my job and running, I kept myself busy. I looked forward to moving into our new house, still under construction, that Joy and I found during our second trip to Ann Arbor. Located in a neighboring township, the house was 20 minutes from my office and 10 minutes from downtown. Only half a mile further in the opposite direction from downtown the landscape changed from large housing developments to farms and dirt roads, a perfect surface for long-distance running. Our new house was located in a golf-course community. Although neither Joy nor I golfed, we liked that the development was big enough to go for long walks—something Joy and I had enjoyed doing together for as long as we had known each other—without having to worry about traffic. Also, there were plenty of kids in the neighborhood and we had a large, flat back yard, an ideal place for Alan and Sam to play.

The transition was difficult, but not nearly as hard as Joy and I had feared. Alan, showing remarkable resilience, made two friends within the first week at his new school—although it took at least a year to get over the loss he experienced from moving away from his friends in

Amherst. Meanwhile, Joy enrolled Sam in a pre-K program for children with learning disabilities—Sam qualified by virtue of his ADHD. After spending a few weeks unpacking and getting settled, Joy started looking for a job. Her search lasted less than two weeks; she accepted an offer she thought she would love at the first place she interviewed.

Marathon Maniac

I hadn't given so much as a thought to running another marathon...until I moved to Ann Arbor. The move meant a reunion with my old friend and running partner, Jim, now a professor at University of Michigan's business school. After I arrived there, Jim and I started doing long runs together on Sunday mornings. He had run the Chicago Marathon in October and had qualified for Boston—the goal of every recreational marathon runner. After hearing Jim's story a few times, I became nostalgic and before I knew it I had caught the marathon bug again. When Jim wasn't around I did the long runs on my own. I didn't know yet where and when I would run my next marathon. But that didn't matter. For the time being just getting into shape and enjoying the long runs was all I needed.

Once I got into marathon running again I got in all the way. Within a few weeks, Jim and I had increased the distance of our long runs to fifteen miles. After Joy and the boys arrived in Ann Arbor in January, I set my sights on the 2002 Detroit Marathon for the following fall. In the past, I had never given much thought as to how best to train for a marathon. I would just increase the distance of my long run, get comfortable running that distance at a good pace, increase the distance of my long run some more and repeat. Jim, on the other hand, was well read on the subject of training. He approached most things in a thoughtful, meticulous manner and had read numerous articles on how to train. He explained to me that a marathon training regimen should include a mix of long, *slow* runs; hard medium-length runs, called tempo runs; and speed workouts on a track. After initially insisting that my approach worked for me, I saw Jim was right and started training for the Detroit Marathon the right way.

I started doing speed work-outs in early summer. The University of Michigan has a top-of-the-line outdoor track that at that time was open to the public whenever the track team wasn't using it. The track was located about a ten-minute drive from my office at MedStat. I started doing my speed workouts there every Tuesday evening with the Ann Arbor Track Club, but I found the track too crowded, the workout too short, and AATC members too clique-y, so I switched to Wednesdays. I almost always worked out by myself, but every once in a while someone else would be on the track at the same time and we would strike up a conversation, agreeing to do part of our work-outs together.

One day a guy who introduced himself as Wally joined me for one of my quarter mile reps. Despite being about ten years older than me, Wally was much faster. He said he had seen me working out and told me he was impressed I had the motivation to do these workouts by myself. He said there was a running group that got together on Wednesdays that had some really great people in it and suggested I ask if I could join them.

I had no way of knowing it at the time, but I learned later that Wally was one of the top runners in the Ann Arbor area for his age group. As for his tip on the running group, I thanked him, but didn't intend to try to hook up with them. I felt I had a pretty good routine and didn't want to change it. It would be a few months before I saw Wally again.

The Detroit Marathon finished on the 50-yard line of the Lions' Ford Field, which I reached in a less than spectacular time of 3:37:38. (I have the exact times for all the races I have run since moving to Ann Arbor because they are posted on the Web.) Although disappointed, I knew I would have plenty of other opportunities to run another marathon, so I quickly got over my disappointment.

Boston or Bust

It's a good thing I did because Jim and Don were talking about running the Boston Marathon in April 2003 and I wanted to join them. Running the Boston Marathon had been a dream of mine since high school. Also, I would see Don for the first time in several years. Joy and I decided that she and the kids would come and we would make a mini vacation of it.

There was only one problem. A big part of the allure of the Boston Marathon is that it is the only U.S. marathon besides the Olympic trials that has a qualifying time to get in. Jim and Don had qualified, but I still needed to run a sub-3:30 marathon. I did a Google search and found the Houston Marathon in January. Houston would be easy to get to and at least the airfare would be free, since I could use my frequent flyer miles.

I had a serious mishap about two months before the race that almost caused me to miss it. Jim and I had started a long run in late afternoon and by the time we were close to finishing it had gotten dark. I tripped over a speed table and landed flush on my left shoulder. The pain was excruciating. Jim went to the nearest house for help and thankfully they let him in so he could call his wife, Sue. A few minutes later Sue picked us up and rushed me to the hospital. I had broken my clavicle.

A couple of days later I saw my primary care physician. She told me to hold off on running for a few weeks to give my clavicle some time to heal. But I couldn't bring myself to do that. I needed to qualify for Boston. I ran for the first time just one week after the accident and two weeks after the accident I ran eighteen miles. During that run my shoulder hurt like hell, but so did my legs. I kept going, telling myself it must be okay to run that far because my legs were hurting every bit as much as my shoulder and there was nothing wrong with my legs. Needless to say, my logic was twisted, but I was obsessed about getting to run in Boston. A few weeks later, I ran the Houston Marathon in 3:25:19; not great, but good enough to qualify.

After so much anticipation, my Boston Marathon experience was a major disappointment. I dropped out less than half-way through. Early in the race I found it difficult to keep up even an eight minute per mile pace. Something was definitely wrong—even on my worst days I could run at this pace effortlessly for several miles. At 12 p.m., the starting time, it was warm but not warm enough to have been a factor this early in the race. By the five-mile mark I could barely lift my legs. Adding to the strangeness of the situation was that I wasn't especially tired. By about the nine-mile mark I could barely run at all. I would stop to walk, feel okay and try to run again, but would not be able to move my legs. I dropped out when I saw a medical tent at the twelve-mile mark.

I felt guilty for not finishing but I knew that dropping out was my only option. What would have been the point of trying to walk the remaining twelve and a half miles? I'd proven in Newport that I could will myself to keep going no matter how badly I felt. But this time I didn't feel much pain. I just couldn't move my legs.

I now think an early episode of Parkinson's was the main culprit. Why, then, did this incident happen at least two years before I had even a clue I had a movement disorder? The best theory is one Joy suggested. I had Parkinson's long before my diagnosis. But I was in such excellent shape, it hadn't become apparent. Running three marathons within six months and running around the day before with my kids was just enough to tip the balance and make my Parkinson's noticeable on that day.

By the time I got back to Ann Arbor, I didn't feel quite as badly about my performance anymore. I had my chance to run in the Boston Marathon and it didn't work out the way I expected. But so what! At least I was still healthy. There would be plenty more marathons in my future and I was ready to move on to the next one. In fact, my next running adventure had already begun.

The Group

Ann Arbor is not known as a hotbed for running, and yet it has numerous groups, some with very good runners.

Many of these runners do not have an official name—they are just a group of people that get together to run on a regular basis. Shortly after my trip to Boston I had the good fortune to join one of these.

The University of Michigan has an excellent indoor track facility located just across the parking lot from the outdoor track. Having run less than twelve miles of the Boston Marathon, I didn't need my normal three to four weeks to recover. Nine days after the marathon on a Wednesday evening, I went to the indoor track to resume my speed workouts.

As I jogged around the track for my warm-ups, a group of about fifteen runners sped by me on the inside lane. They passed me three more times before they stopped to rest. A man who appeared to be in his mid-sixties called out each runner's splits as they went by. He occasionally offered a word or two of encouragement but did not raise his voice or goad anyone to run faster.

No more than three minutes later they started up again. When they passed me on their first lap around the track, I noticed a man near the back of the pack who looked familiar. But seeing only his back as he motored past me, I couldn't place him. I turned around so that the next time he passed me I would be able to see his face. This time I recognized him immediately—it was Wally, the guy who had befriended me the previous fall. He came over during the next rest period and told me what I had already surmised—this was the running group he had told me about last fall. He invited me to join the work out. Before I had a chance to ask him whether he was sure it was okay, he said, "Don't worry about it; I will let Bill know." Then he dashed off to where the man who had been calling out the times stood. They talked for a few seconds and then Bill nodded his approval. A minute later I lined up with the group as they started their next interval.

It became immediately apparent to me after we started that the people in this group ran fast, much faster than they appeared to be running when I watched them from the sidelines. I finished last, a stride behind the next slowest runner and several seconds behind Wally.

Despite my last-place finish, Bill and the other runners made me feel welcome. Bill called out my splits just as he did for everyone else. As we lined up for my second interval, Seanna, the fastest woman in the group, introduced herself to me and asked me for my name. Then she told me she was glad I could join the workout, turned around and took off as we started the next interval. I showed up the next Wednesday and the Wednesday after that. Before long I felt accepted as a regular member of the group.

After my fourth workout with them, The Group, as I began referring to them, moved its workouts outdoors. We met every Wednesday at 5:15. I normally did not leave my office until six or six-thirty, frequently attending meetings late in the day. But I let it be known to everyone, including my boss, that I would no longer be available on Wednesdays after five.

When I visited Ann Arbor for my first job interview with MedStat, I expected the area to be flat. And indeed, the biggest hill I saw on the trip back and forth from the airport to MedStat's building was the on-ramp to the highway. Little did I know that Ann Arbor is actually very hilly in places, especially near the Huron River. Also, as I discovered when Joy and I went house hunting, you don't have to go far from downtown Ann Arbor to find rural areas with mostly dirt roads. Hill running is a great way to build strength and dirt roads are a great surface for long distance running. The Group met at a parking lot on Huron River Drive, right next to the river, and did most of its workouts on the nearby dirt roads.

The outdoor workouts can best be described as brutal. I vividly remember my first outdoor workout with The Group. We started with a two and a half mile warm-up run over a route that had several large hills. The warm-up run started slowly enough, but we gradually sped up. By the time we got about two-thirds of the way through the warm-up, we were running at about a 7:15 per mile pace—way too fast for me. I had to slow down. But I couldn't slow down too much. I had to keep the last person in front of me in sight so I would know where we were going. I arrived at the starting point for the actual workout feeling like I already had done a workout. Fortunately, I had enough time to rest before the real workout began.

We began by running "at speed" for a quarter mile up an incredibly steep hill, jogging back down and, without stopping, repeating until we had run up the hill four times. Then, after about a five-minute rest, we ran a mile at speed, rested again, and ran another mile at speed. We then did the same thing, but in the opposite direction, finishing the fourth mile at the top of the huge hill. The workout ended with a jog down the hill and one last run back up, at speed. I don't know how I was able to do the warm-down run back to the parking lot, but somehow I made it, well after the rest of The Group.

Exhausted, but elated, I was already looking forward to the next workout by the time I got into my car. I had pushed myself to the limit and there was no better feeling for me than that. I could hardly wait until the next Wednesday when I would get to do it again.

Losing My Gait

In retrospect it should have been obvious, but hindsight is always 20/20. The Parkinson's Foundation lists ten early warning signs of Parkinson's Disease and for at least ten years before my diagnosis I had four of them: loss of smell, trouble sleeping, constipation, and stooping or hunching over. Joy and Jim noticed the fifth, masked face, about four years before my diagnosis. Each of these signs appeared to have a separate cause. They were random observations in a sea of data. Unaware that these signs were in any way connected, I never reported them all at once to any of my doctors.

Running provided its own clues. The first hint that something might be wrong came in October 2003, two weeks before my second Detroit Marathon. Thirteen miles into a slow fourteen-mile run—my last long run before the race—I started to have a strange feeling of losing my gait. The left and right sides of my body seemed to have fallen out of sync with each other. I tried to compensate by concentrating on my stride, but the feeling grew more intense. I felt almost as if I had forgotten how to run as I struggled to put one foot in front of the other. After about a minute I had to stop. I walked for a few minutes and then tried running again. Thankfully, the gait problem went away. I jogged slowly the rest of the way home.

I was perplexed about what had just happened, but not alarmed. I had experienced all manner of aches and pains during my marathon training but never had a serious injury. Usually whatever pain I felt dissipated within a few weeks of running the marathon. I had no reason to believe this gait problem would be any different. I didn't give it another thought. The incident soon receded into memory.

Two weeks later I finished the Detroit Marathon in 3:21:24, just off my goal of 3:20. By most objective standards I had run an outstanding race—I finished above the ninetieth percentile for my age group and beat the Boston Marathon qualifying time for my age group by eight and a half minutes. But I was not satisfied. I knew I could beat 3:20 and thought I had a chance to go under 3:15. I couldn't wait to get back to training for my next marathon.

By now I had become a hard-core, two-marathons-a-year running junkie. I trained year round. The only times I did not train were during the tapering before a marathon and the recovery afterward. Running had once again become more than just an avocation; it had become a lifestyle. Within a few days of running the Detroit Marathon I decided on St. Louis 2004 for my next marathon.

The second sign that something might be wrong came after I had reached twenty miles for my long runs during training for St. Louis. On several occasions, near the end of these runs, I found myself leaning backwards and to my left, as if someone had come from behind me, grabbed my left shoulder and gently pulled me backwards. I compensated by shortening my stride and leaning forward slightly. After two or three minutes the feeling abated to the point where I could resume my normal stride. The same thing happened several more times and each time I regained my normal stride within a few minutes. I attributed these incidents to fatigue and didn't think much more about them. I ran the marathon without incident, finishing with a time of 3:22:13.

I took my usual three to four weeks off to recover and then started training again, this time for the 2004 Detroit Marathon. Early in my training cycle, before I started putting in the heavy miles, I ran a couple of short races. I did well, averaging 6:30 per mile for a four-mile race and 7:00 per mile for a 10K. I won my age group for the 10k.

I followed my usual practice of gradually increasing the distance of my long Sunday runs. As I neared the end of my first sixteen-mile run I felt the same odd sensation of falling backwards and to my left that I had felt the previous spring. Only this time the feeling was stronger. The same thing happened the following Sunday, and the Sunday after that. These episodes concerned me, but I always recovered my gait within a few minutes and never had to stop. So I brushed my concerns aside.

I woke up the morning of the Detroit Marathon feeling good but not great. Still, having come so close the last two times, I thought I had a reasonably good chance to finally break the 3:20 barrier. But this was not to be my day. Just three miles into the race I found myself straining to maintain a 7:30 per mile pace. The strain became an out and out struggle when I reached the Ambassador Bridge to Canada and began the long uphill climb to the midpoint of the expanse. Not wanting to expend too much energy this early in the race, I slowed down. Then I let myself go during the downhill portion. I hoped that after running a fast downhill mile, a 7:30 per mile pace would feel relatively slow.

This tactic did not work. I soon found it more difficult to run 7:30 miles than I had before crossing the bridge. Realizing I had no chance to achieve my 3:20 goal, I slowed down to a comfortable pace. I considered dropping out at the halfway point, but decided to keep running. I finished in 3:49, frustrated and confused about why the race had gone so badly. I didn't experience the gait problem, but my legs had felt heavy from the start of the race. Why?

Unable to answer this question, I chalked up my performance to just having a bad day. This had happened before—in Boston, for example—and would probably happen again, I told myself. Despite my adherence to a strict training regimen, I never knew how well I would run on any given day until I started running.

My frustration and disappointment did not last long, though. I trained as hard as I did because I enjoyed it. My Wednesday evening workouts with the running group were the highlight of my week. I also looked forward to a long run every Sunday. Whereas most people who trained hard did so to achieve a goal, I set goals for myself to justify training so hard. With that in mind, I looked forward to my next marathon.

I set my sight next on the spring 2005 Glass City Marathon in Toledo, Ohio. I thought this would be the ideal race for me. With about a thousand participants, it promised to be less crowded at the start than the big city marathons, the course was mostly flat, and Toledo was less than an hour's drive from home. Toledo had one other thing going for it, as well—it was the site of my greatest triumph as a runner. In 1981, I ran the Toledo Heart-Watchers marathon in 2:54:32. I hoped that some of the karma from that day would spill over and help me to succeed this time.

Initially my training went well. But then, when I reached fourteen miles for my long run, the gait problem came roaring back. It occurred more often and with greater intensity than it had the previous fall. With increasing frequency I had to stop and walk for ten to fifteen seconds before I could recover my gait. I soon became accustomed to losing my gait during long runs.

I told Joy about the gait problem and, concerned but not alarmed, she suggested I see my doctor about it. I told her I would—after the marathon. I had not yet connected the dots between my recent gait problem and the one-time loss-of-gait incident that occurred two weeks before the 2003 Detroit Marathon. Nor did I have any inkling that these events might be related in any way to the tired legs I experienced during the Boston Marathon and the 2004 Detroit Marathon. Despite having to stop every so often during long runs, training was going well. I sensed something might be wrong, but not wanting to believe it, I continued working out harder than ever. Simply put, I was in a state of denial.

Then, during one of my tempo runs, I felt a wave of numbness course up from my right foot through my body and to my head as I landed. The numbness, not unlike a shock from static electricity, lasted less than a second. I had almost forgotten about it until a few weeks later when Jim joined me for the first half of a twenty-two-mile distance run. Less than a mile into the run I experienced the same thing, this time after I landed on my left foot. I asked Jim whether he had ever experienced anything similar. He looked at me incredulously. He said no, he had never experienced numbness while running, it was not normal and I really should see a doctor about it. I told Jim the same thing I had told Joy—I was too busy now but would schedule a doctor visit after the marathon.

The real reason I put off seeing my doctor was that I was afraid she would tell me to curtail or possibly even stop running. I had begun to worry that maybe my gait problem and the two recent numbness incidents were signs of a neurological disorder. I desperately wanted to take a shot at breaking 3:20 because I feared this might be my last opportunity.

Race day for the Glass City Marathon finally came. I was in terrific shape and had slept well the night before. With temperatures expected to get no higher than the mid-fifties, conditions were ideal. I had some nagging doubts about whether and how the gait problem would affect my performance, but I was able to push these aside. Ready to finally run my sub-3:20 marathon, I couldn't wait for the race to begin.

It could not possibly have gone worse. I started out comfortably running the 7:30 per mile pace that I had established as my goal. But within five miles my gait problem reared its ugly head. I walked for about ten seconds and was able to start running again, but less than a mile later the gait problem returned. I tried several more times to run, but each time the problem came on more quickly. By the time I approached the ten-mile mark, I was able to run no more than a couple of hundred yards at a time before having to stop and walk again. I knew then that this race was over and suspected my life as a marathon runner was, as well.

During the drive back to Ann Arbor, I vowed that first thing Monday morning I would make an appointment to see my doctor. An eighteen-month odyssey that finally resulted in my being diagnosed with Parkinson's had begun.

CHAPTER 16
I'M A PARKIE NOW

The Mayo Clinic website defines Parkinson's Disease (PD) as "a progressive disorder of the nervous system that affects movement." This loss of movement is caused by inability of the brain to produce dopamine. The disease is notoriously difficult to diagnose. Dopamine deficiency cannot be detected by a blood test, CT scan, MRI, or other advanced test.

The National Parkinson's Disease Foundation lists ten early warning signs of PD:

- Tremor or shaking
- Small handwriting
- Loss of smell
- Trouble sleeping
- Trouble moving or walking
- Constipation
- A soft or low voice
- Masked face
- Dizziness or fainting
- Stooping or hunching over

It would be easy for doctors to identify their PD patients if all of them presented with these ten signs. But Parkies rarely experience these changes in that way. Each person is unique. At the early stages of PD, most patients are probably aware of only three or four of these signs. But neither they nor their doctors connect the dots. To make matters more complicated, patients often complain about other conditions that have nothing to do with PD.

. . . .

And so my odyssey proceeded in its own unique fashion. As I promised myself during the drive home from the Toledo Glass City Marathon, I called my primary care physician, who I will henceforth refer to as Dr. G, at eight a.m. Monday morning. I had no reason to be nervous about making this call, but I was. My problems were difficult to describe—and they kept changing from week to week. The imaginary man pulling me back from my left shoulder had moved on to ruin somebody else's gait. Now, whenever I ran, I felt like I was running in waist-deep water. I wasn't necessarily tired. I just couldn't get my legs to move. I used to be faster than Jim. Now I could no longer beat him even when he ran backwards.

I had on and off lower back pain. Also, far more painful, if I landed on my right heel the wrong way, I felt an excruciating jab, like someone slicing a knife from one side of the heel to the other. I had felt pain similar to the heel and back pain before, after two previous marathons. Both times it took two weeks to get an appointment with Dr. G and both times my pain had diminished by the time I saw her. When I finally got into Dr. G's office, she asked me four or five questions, pressed my back and heel, and then said with a smirk, "If you stopped running so much you would be fine."

I wondered what would happen this time. Would she take me seriously? The only thing new this time was my gait problem. Dr. G did take me seriously. She told me I had a neurologic disorder and she would need to refer me to a neurologist.

· · · · · · · · ·

I am lucky to live in a place where the best of care is available. Dr. G referred me to the University of Michigan Health System (UMHS), one of the top medical research institutions in the country. Many of the physicians I saw there are highly specialized. They all seemed to be genuinely interested in trying to help me.

During the year and a half it took to diagnose me, I saw a bevy of doctors who subjected me to numerous tests, including blood and urine tests, MRIs, CAT scans, and MRGs, to name a few.

At times I worried they might not continue to take me seriously. I imagined them in a conference, saying, *Nothing we try on this guy works. Also, he keeps changing his story. First he complains about his lower back and a sharp pain in his heel if he lands wrong, plus a gait change when he runs. Now he no longer mentions his back or heel, but has added running through waist-deep water to his list of complaints. Is this guy just making it up?*

But through the entire ordeal, they took me seriously. Only once, early on in the process, did a doctor jokingly suggest I limit my runs to sixteen miles.

After eighteen long months, it took an observant neurology intern's epiphany to diagnose my Parkinson's. She noted a slight tremor in my right hand I had not yet noticed myself. Then, thinking it might be PD, she ran down the list of signs, asking which were relevant for me. I had all of them. On November 21, 2006, my neurologist, Dr. L, gave me my diagnosis. I had Parkinson's.

I have learned a few lessons through this experience. First: we're all different and our signs and symptoms may vary; the disease progression rate is not the same for everyone; and different medications are required in varying doses depending on the individual. Also, since PD is generally a disease of the elderly, other diseases often accompany it, complicating efforts to diagnose the disorder.

The second lesson is that doctors don't know everything. The best physicians understand and accept that. For example, I have come to understand that my PD and peripheral neuropathy (PN) are related to each other and extra Sinemet (a PD medication) helps to relieve some of the PN pain. One younger and rather arrogant doctor said it was impossible for PD and PN to work in cahoots, but another explained how it might happen and endorsed using Sinemet for PN pain relief.

. . . .

There are many excellent memoirs that track the course of the disease of a loved one or the author as PD takes its toll. I chose to take a different approach, focusing instead on my spiritual and intellectual life with PD.

Although I have described some of the medical specifics, I would like to focus on what I feel is more compelling: questions universal to those diagnosed with progressive degenerative diseases. *Why me? How do I deal with this disease? How do I make the best of it? How can I make a positive difference while I still have the physical strength and cognitive capabilities largely intact? How long will it last? How has it changed my life? Were any changes for the better? How do I make a difference in the time I have left? What legacy, if any, will I leave?*

The road to diagnosis is different for everyone, but once individuals have been diagnosed, the questions are the same.

· · · · · · · · ·

Although I did not want this memoir to be a day-to-day accounting of my medical condition, I realized I needed to give readers some indication of how far my disease had progressed at each point in my narrative. I hadn't kept a diary, so I wondered how I would add this all-important context to my thoughts and feelings. I needed markers to describe my physical status at various points in the narrative.

Thankfully, my disability insurance company, which we will call Acme to protect the innocent and not-so-innocent, came to the rescue. Despite the fact that my diseases are progressive and so can only get worse, every eighteen months Acme requires me and my doctor to complete a long questionnaire describing my physical and cognitive capabilities. They ask four open-ended questions, some with follow-up questions, which for the sake of brevity I paraphrase here.

1. Please describe your current medical condition or conditions. Also, describe any changes that have occurred in the last 18 months.

2. Please list all the types of activities you do during the course of a typical day. What do you do specifically from the time you arise in the morning until you retire at night?

3. For each condition causing your disability, indicate the activities of daily living for which you need help. Describe the help you need.

4. What kinds of hobbies or social/community activities did you engage in prior to your disability and what do you engage in now?

I spent hours working on my responses, making sure I described the nuances of my condition and why they prevented me from working. After completing the most recent questionnaire I saw that my answers gave as complete a description of my medical condition as anything else I could imagine myself writing. So I decided to use these questionnaires as the markers, which describe my health status at relevant points in time. Thank you, Acme.

In February 2009 I applied for disability compensation when I reduced my hours from forty to thirty-two per week. At that time I'd had many forms to fill out for my employer, but had not yet needed to fill out any for the insurance company. When I reduced my hours, Acme required only a statement from my neurologist, shown on these pages.

ATTENDING PHYSICIAN'S STATEMENT OF FUNCTIONALITY
To be completed by the Employee

Patient Name: Ira Fried   Social Security Number: ____   Date of Birth: ____

Employer's Name: Thomson Reuters

I hereby authorize release of information on this form by the below named physician for the purpose of claim processing.

Signed (Patient): Ira Fried   Date: 2/24/09

To be completed by the Attending Physician - Use current information from your patient's most recent office visit or examination to complete this form. *(The patient is responsible for the completion of this form without expense to the Company)*

Patient's condition is a result of: [x] Sickness [ ] Injury [ ] Pregnancy

If pregnancy, What is the expected delivery date? ____

Is condition due to illness or injury that is work related? [ ] Yes [x] No

DIAGNOSIS

Primary diagnosis: PARKINSON'S DISEASE   ICD-9 Code: 332.0

Secondary diagnosis(es): FATIGUE   ICD-9 Code(s): 780.7

Current Subjective symptoms: FATIGUE, SLOWNESS

Physical Examination Findings: RIGHT HAND TREMOR, SLOWNESS OF GAIT AND MOVEMENT

Blood pressure: 136/84   Date BP taken: 2/24/09   Height: 73.5 (IN) Weight: 215.5 LBS

Current Pertinent Test Results (list all results, or enclose test result reports):

Test: ____ Date: ____ Results: ____

Test: ____ Date: ____ Results: ____

Current Medications, Dosage and Frequency: REQUIP 4MG PO TID, SINEMET 25/100 2 PILLS PO TID

TREATMENT PLAN

Current Treatment Plan: CONTINUE CURRENT MEDICATIONS

What is the Frequency / Duration of Treatment? EVERY 3 MONTHS   Date(s) of Treatment: ____

First Office Visit for this condition: 1/21/06   Last Office Visit: 2/24/09   Next Scheduled Office Visit: ____

Date patient reported stopping work: 3/6/09   Date of disability: 11/21/06   Expected return to work date: ____

Has patient been referred to any other physician? [ ] Yes [x] No If "Yes," Date of Referral(s): ____

Referral Physician Name: ____ Phone Number: ( ) ____ Specialty: ____

Has surgery been performed since last report? [ ] Yes [x] No Is surgery planned? [ ] Yes [ ] No

If "Yes," on what date(s): ____ Procedure(s): ____ CPT Code: ____

Was patient hospitalized since last report? [ ] Yes [x] No If "Yes," Hospital Name: ____

Phone Number: ( ) ____ Admission Date: ____ Discharge Date: ____

LC-7135-2 [FI] Printed in U.S.A.   Page 1 of 2   01/2008

FUNCTIONAL CAPABILITIES

Please complete the applicable portion of this section based on your most recent assessment.

In a general workplace environment the patient is able to:

	Sit	Stand	Walk
Number of hours at a time	8	1	0.5
Total hours/day	8	1	1

Please check the frequency with which the patient can perform the following activities:

R = Right L = Left B = Bilateral		Never	Occasionally (1-33%)	Frequently (34-67%)	No Restrictions	Not Applicable
Lift / carry 1 to 10 lbs.		R L B	R L (B)	R L B	R L B	
Lift / carry 11 to 20 lbs.		R L B	R L (B)	R L B	R L B	
Lift / carry 21 to 50 lbs.		R L (B)	R L B	R L B	R L B	
Lift / carry 51 to 100 lbs.		R L (B)	R L B	R L B	R L B	
Lift / carry over 100 lbs.		R L (B)	R L B	R L B	R L B	
Bending at waist			✓			
Kneeling / crouching		✓				
Driving				✓		
Reaching only (not load-bearing)	Above shoulder	R L B	R L B	R L B	R L (B)	
	At waist / desk level	R L B	R L B	R L B	R L (B)	
	Below waist / desk level	R L B	R L B	R L B	R L (B)	
Fingering / handling		R L B	R L B	R L (B)	R L B	

Is the patient's vision impaired? ☐ Yes ☑ No   If "Yes," please describe the extent of the impairment _____

Best corrected visual acuity: R _____ L _____   Hand dominance: ☐ R ☐ L

Does the patient have a psychiatric / cognitive impairment? ☐ Yes ☑ No   If "Yes," please describe the extent of the impairment and its etiology: _____

Expected duration of any current restriction(s) or limitation(s) listed above: LIFETIME

Do you believe the patient is competent to endorse checks and direct the use of the proceeds? ☑ Yes ☐ No

Can the patient participate in vocational rehabilitation services (this may include worksite accommodations, identifying alternative work, and or retraining assistance)? ☑ Yes ☐ No If "No," anticipated date they can participate: _____

PHYSICIAN INFORMATION

Provider's Name: _____		Telephone Number: _____
Degree: MD	Specialty: NEUROLOGY	Fax Number: _____
License Number: _____	Social Security Number or EIN _____	
Street Address: _____	City: ANN ARBOR	State: MI Zip Code: 48109
Signature: _____		Date signed: 2/24/02

CHAPTER 17
MY LIFE AS A PARKIE

What's the Big Deal?

People sometimes ask me how I felt when I learned I had Parkinson's. Did I get angry? Depressed? The truth is I did not feel either of these emotions. More than anything else I felt a palpable sense of relief. Finally I had an explanation for my running problems. The diagnosis also explained some other things I had just begun to notice, like the slight tremor in my right hand and the tendency for my handwriting to become very small.

I reacted to my diagnosis by going into planning mode, as I usually do when something bad happens. I made a mental list of the things I had to do. I put telling my family and close friends at the top of the list. I decided to call Edythe first because she was the person in my family I was closest to; I also thought she would take the news calmly and with empathy. I procrastinated for a few days until Joy finally ordered me to make the call. As I punched in the numbers, Joy sat beside me to provide support in case I needed it. I didn't think I did.

Edythe picked up the phone and said, "Hello Brother."

Without wasting any time, I gave her the news—I had been diagnosed with Parkinson's.

She started to cry. I tried to reassure her it was no big deal, but she continued crying for another minute or so until she said she could no longer stay on the phone. Perplexed, I held the phone next to my ear for a few seconds after she hung up.

I asked Joy why Edythe had gotten so upset.

Joy nodded knowingly. "Parkinson's is a serious disease."

Having seen numerous Parkinson's patients during her career as a speech and language pathologist, Joy knew all too well what problems PD might cause. In addition to the symptoms that Dr. L had noticed when she made the diagnosis, I could expect to experience difficulty swallowing, voice-softening to the point where it could compromise communication, slow movement and rigid muscles, impaired balance, which might lead to falls, bladder problems, including an inability to urinate, pain, and scariest of all, loss of cognitive abilities, possibly leading to dementia. And this was only a partial list. My doctors could not predict which maladies would affect me. Each Parkie experiences PD differently. Joy knew all this but did not elaborate. Dr. L had given me all I needed to comprehend that PD is a very big deal. I just needed to review this information at my own pace.

Only six days after my diagnosis, I was better off staying in my state of denial. My reaction to the Parkinson's diagnosis was not unusual for me. I responded in much the same way upon learning that my father had died suddenly at age fifty-one of a massive heart attack. Joy and I were living in Chicago when he died, but I was in Connecticut on a business trip. After eating dinner with colleagues, I returned to my room to find the message light on my phone flashing. It was Joy telling me I needed to call Lony right away. I called and Lony gave me the news. At first I felt nothing. Instead, my mind focused on the logistics of getting to New York the next morning. Once I had worked that out I went for a long walk. I thought about my relationship with my father—it had improved greatly in the last year after a tumultuous adolescence and early adulthood. Then my thoughts turned to the financial impact my father's death would have on my mother. For the last ten years his alimony payments had been her primary means of support. *What will happen now*, I worried. *What will I need to do to help her? Am I responsible for her?*

I wanted to grieve for my father. I tried to cry. But I couldn't. I remained devoid of normal human emotion through the memorial service and funeral, even as I poured the ceremonial first shovel of dirt on my father's grave. Not until three days later did I feel any emotion. Without warning, I started bawling uncontrollably. I continued for perhaps five minutes and then stopped.

A few weeks later I had a vivid dream in which my father and I played a closely contested tennis match. I could see he didn't look well but I kept pressing on, determined to beat him. As I won the final point he crumpled to the ground. I had caused his heart attack! I woke up in a cold sweat, screaming. Since then I have had many dreams about my father, all of them positive—in most of these dreams he has given me advice on an issue I was struggling with at the time.

I think I inherited this tendency to defer emotions, both positive and negative, from my father. He never seemed to get flustered when something really bad happened. I expected him to fly into a rage when I brought home a report card full of Cs, Ds, and Fs in eighth grade. But nothing happened. He reacted with complete calm. After looking over the report card he returned it to me and, without a hint of anger in his voice, told me he would let me know later what the appropriate punishment would be. On the other hand, my father often lost his cool over the smallest provocations. I recall numerous incidents when my father got into heated arguments with gas station attendants or toll collectors over minor infractions he thought they committed.

I can recall feeling intense, unbridled emotion immediately after a major event only a few times in my life. The first time was the punch-in-the-gut anguish I felt when my father told me he and my mother had broken up. The second was the overwhelming love I felt for Alan when he was born a healthy baby after Joy's first three pregnancies had ended in miscarriage. I felt the same rush of love for Sam when he was born after two additional miscarriages. But this time I felt none of those emotions. I went right into planning mode.

· · · · · · · · ·

First, Joy and I needed to talk to Alan and Sam. We decided to tell them, then thirteen and ten, as matter-of-factly as we could that I had Parkinson's. We gave them the *Reader's Digest* version of what we knew about the disease, assured them everything was going to be okay, and then ask them if they had any questions. I had been concerned about how they might react, but the meeting turned out to be anticlimactic. They listened to what Joy and I had to say, asked a few questions and then, apparently satisfied that my illness would not have much impact on their lives, asked if they could go back to what they were doing. Although Joy and I knew more must be going on in their minds than they were willing to reveal, we were relieved they had taken the news well.

Next was learning about my rights under Thomson Reuter's (MedStat) disability policy and the Americans with Disabilities Act. Unsure of whether and how I should inform my employer of my illness, I hired an attorney to advise me. She confirmed what I remembered from the employee rights training session I had recently attended. The Americans with Disabilities Act protected me from discrimination due to my illness and required my employer to make reasonable accommodations for me.

I told her I had an excellent working relationship with my boss and I was in good standing with senior management. I also told her that, to the best of my knowledge, Thomson Reuters had always treated its employees fairly.

Armed with this information, she drafted an email for me to send to Marjorie, my boss, and Human Resources, notifying them of my illness. She corroborated my interpretation of the disability insurance policies. She verified that both the standard and supplemental policies would pay partial benefits if I needed to reduce my hours. And most important, she validated my assessment that the two policies combined would pay enough for my family to maintain our current standard of living should I need to go on full disability. With these issues resolved, I knew I would not have to worry about my family's financial future. I was lucky these policies were made available to me and I could take advantage of them. Working through the legal and financial ramifications of my illness was not difficult. I handled it just like a dozen other projects I typically had going at work at any given time, checking off action items as I completed them. Coping with the physical realities of Parkinson's, and beginning a couple of years later, also peripheral neuropathy, presented an entirely different challenge. I could not create a project to make this problem go away.

Living with a progressive, incurable condition like Parkinson's is, as the Bob Seger song goes, like "Running Against the Wind." With Parkinson's the wind never stops blowing. And no matter which direction you turn, it is always a headwind—a headwind that grows imperceptibly but inexorably stronger with each passing day.

For the first couple of years after my diagnosis, 2007 and 2008, living with Parkinson's felt more like running into a light breeze than a strong headwind. It affected my running, but not much else. During the height of my marathon-running days, a few years earlier, I had run outdoors seven days a week without any regard for the weather or road conditions. I did this not because I didn't like any other types of exercise, but because I didn't want to upset my marathon training schedule. By the time I received my Parkinson's diagnosis, I had given up running marathons and, as a result, had become less compulsive about running. I no longer ran outside on cold winter days. Instead, I exercised indoors using the elliptical cycle Joy had bought me as a birthday present. I also began riding my bicycle during the warmer months. As running became increasingly difficult, I started using my bike more often. By 2008, bicycling had replaced running as my primary mode of exercise. I mapped out several routes and became every bit as maniacal about trying to better my times on these routes as I had been on my running loops. I rarely ran anymore but I still thought of myself as a runner.

The breeze had become stronger by early spring 2009. After a winter of working out exclusively indoors, I tried to go for a run the first nice day in March. To my surprise, I couldn't finish my easy five-mile recovery run without stopping several times to walk. Also, my pace had slowed to more than ten minutes a mile. Over the next two to three weeks I tried to run several more times, each time with the same result. I realized then that my days as a runner had ended.

I cannot fathom why that did not upset me more. It should have been a momentous occasion for me—I used to tell Joy, not entirely joking, to just kill me when I could no longer run. I guess my rational, analytical side must have taken over. I reasoned I could continue to work out every day using my elliptical cycle during the winter and riding a bike the rest of the year. Having found other activities to replace running mitigated the loss I might otherwise have felt. Although no longer a runner, I could still think of myself as an athlete.

I accepted not being able to run as my new normal. But soon, a new problem arose. I began to feel my energy wane in the early afternoons. Accustomed for my entire career to working at full speed until at least six p.m., I now found it difficult to keep up the pace beyond about three. To compensate, I switched from decaf to regular coffee and, in the early afternoon, added a twenty-ounce bottle of Diet Pepsi to the forty-plus ounces I typically drank during lunch. The extra caffeine helped me to power through the afternoon, but now I had to push myself to stay productive.

At the same time I started feeling a strange tingling sensation in my left foot, not unlike the feeling you get when your foot "falls asleep." The feeling came and went. It might last for just a few minutes or for as long as an hour. Then it would go away. At first the tingling feeling had no impact on my workouts. But, concerned about this latest development, I made a note to ask my neurologist about it during my upcoming visit in June.

Over the next three months, the tingling feeling gradually grew more intense. It began to occasionally morph into a pain similar to what I remembered feeling as a child when my toes or fingers thawed after a mild case of frostbite. Then I started feeling the same thing in my right foot.

By the time I visited my neurologist, this new malady had transmogrified from curiosity to minor inconvenience to major distraction. My neurologist listened to me recount the symptoms, asked a few clarifying questions and then told me he wanted me to have an EMG. He explained this test would help him to determine whether a nerve disorder, a disease affecting my foot muscles, or something else had triggered the pain.

I looked up EMG on the Web and learned that it typically is done as part of a two-part test: a Nerve Conduction Velocity (NCV) and an Electromyography (EMG). The Johns Hopkins Website describes the NCV as "a test that measures the speed of conduction of an electrical impulse through a nerve." It describes the EMG as "a test that measures muscle response or electrical activity in response to a nerve's stimulation of the muscle."

At the risk of understatement, I would describe these tests as not the most pleasant way to pass the time. During the first part of the test, the NCV, the medical technician subjected me to a series of electrical shocks of increasing strength on various parts of my lower back, legs, and feet. The strongest shocks would have registered at least a six on the ten-point pain scale. But the real fun began when the technician moved on to the EMG. During this test he stuck what appeared to be six-inch-long needles into the same places where he had shocked me. He left each of these needles in for what seemed like hours, until I relaxed the muscle enough for him to get an accurate reading.

The tests turned out to be worth the temporary discomfort. A few days later my neurologist told me I had peripheral neuropathy, a condition that results from damage to the nerves that carry messages back and forth from the brain and spinal cord to the affected area—in my case, my feet. I asked the neurologist if my Parkinson's or Parkinson's medications might have caused the neuropathy and he replied that the two conditions were unrelated. He prescribed a new medication that, for a while, helped to reduce the pain.

By mid-2009, fatigue concerned me far more than foot pain. Starting some time between two and three most afternoons, I felt as if some unknown force had taken over my body, sapping me of energy and leaving me in a state of fevered exhaustion. Joy urged me to slow down. But driven by a need to excel at my job and hoping to get a long-sought-after promotion to Vice President, I did not heed her advice. I continued to fight through the fatigue each afternoon and leave work at my regular time.

I tried hard to hide the fatigue and naively thought I had succeeded until Marjorie brought it up during one of our weekly one-on-one meetings in late 2009. She told me she and most of my colleagues saw my late afternoon struggles and they had become painful for her to watch. She encouraged me to give some thought to how I could change my schedule to make my afternoons less difficult. She also assured me that, after several months of her lobbying and my winning my fourth President's Club Award, she had finally overcome her boss' reservations concerning my promotion. His reluctance stemmed from his belief that I had been too outspoken about my impolitic views on what it took to succeed in sales. This discussion prompted me to finally listen to the advice Joy had started giving me months earlier—I asked to go on partial disability, reducing my official hours from forty to thirty-two per week. Marjorie readily agreed.

A week later Marjorie told me my impending change in status to part-time employee presented a new potential roadblock to promotion. Thomson Reuters had a long-standing policy, she explained, that only full-time employees could be promoted to Vice President. She told me I should begin the paperwork with HR to go on partial disability, while she worked through the bureaucracy to get an exception to Thomson Reuter's promotion policy.

Over the next several weeks, I spent many frustrating hours getting HR to understand and approve the partial disability arrangement while Marjorie spent a comparable amount of time getting approval for an exception to the promotion policy. But by mid-February, we had completed all the necessary paperwork. On March 1, 2010, I officially became the first part-time employee at Thomson Reuters to be promoted to Vice President.

I do not think I can overstate how much this promotion meant to me. With it came new responsibilities. Now client management staff for the entire Health Plan market reported to me and I "owned" the financials for our entire client base. But for me, the promotion was not about having a greater span of control, nor was it about the money. For me the promotion was about recognition and achievement. Since my parents held me back for a second year of kindergarten, I had wanted to play with the big boys and be recognized as their equal. With this promotion, I had finally done that.

Meanwhile, the neuropathy pain grew steadily worse. My neurologist made frequent changes to medications and dosages. Some helped; some did not. But even when they helped, the improvement proved ephemeral. Despite my strong belief in evidence-based medicine, I turned to alternative treatments for relief. I tried Vitamin B supplements, ointments, foot massage, meditation, even acupuncture, but none of these seemed to do more than take the edge off the pain.

This experience gave me an important insight into the medical profession. Despite all the recent advances in medical science, there is still much that doctors don't know. Having spent my entire career in the managed care industry, I had long since stopped putting doctors up on a pedestal. But I expected my own doctors to be able to answer the most basic questions. Since my neuropathy pain started, I have wondered why it always seems to get worse when the Parkinson's medications wear off. I see some of the top Parkinson's and neuropathy specialists in the country at UMHS and even they cannot answer this question.

I Googled the Web and could find only one peer-reviewed article about a small study that links Parkinson's to peripheral neuropathy. None of the major consumer healthcare Websites, for example, WebMD and Mayo-Clinic.com, list Parkinson's and peripheral neuropathy as a cause or symptom of the other. I now understood that the answer to my question simply did not exist within the current body of knowledge. I still sometimes get frustrated by my doctors' inability to answer all my questions, but I no longer reproach them for it. They are only human, after all.

Despite the limitations Parkinson's and peripheral neuropathy imposed on me, the thought of stopping daily workouts never entered my mind. Instead, I looked for ways to improvise. When I could no longer use my elliptical cycle, I went back to using a stationary bike. And when my feet hurt too much to ride a stationary bike for more than fifteen to twenty minutes at a time, I devised a new exercise that didn't put any pressure on my feet. I lay on my back and alternated between bicycle kicks and bench-pressing five-pound weights. I didn't particularly enjoy this new routine, but it did fulfill a need to get my heart pumping and feel the burn of lactic acid in my arms and legs.

Improvising at work proved to be more difficult.

Although I had officially reduced my hours, my workload actually increased. The main culprit: a large implementation project that was not going well. I started leaving work at about two p.m. after going on partial-disability. I went straight home, changed into more casual clothes, and got right into bed. I made up some time by joining conference calls from home. But it wasn't enough. Rather than taking control of the project as I normally would, I became at best an active participant. Marjorie effectively took over my role as the senior person responsible for success of the project. By mid-2010, we both knew we would need to change my role. The light breeze I had first encountered when I started experiencing the symptoms that led to my Parkinson's diagnosis had become a gale-force wind.

I wish I could say I got up every morning, braced myself for the ever-strengthening headwind, and pushed myself just a little bit harder than I did the day before. But I would not have had the willpower to do that. Fortunately, I stumbled upon a better way to cope—denial.

These forms show March 2011 materials related to my application for full-time disability, including a claimant questionnaire and physician's statement from my neurologist. In March 2011 my condition had deteriorated. Fatigue was a big problem. Peripheral neuropathy was just starting, but fatigue continued to be my biggest issue, requiring an application for full disability. The application includes a Claimant Questionnaire that I filled out by hand to describe my condition. At that time I could still write legibly. I attached a typed Addendum adding comments that could not fit on the questionnaire.

3/16/2011

CLAIMANT QUESTIONNAIRE
(Read instructions carefully before completing this form.)

Policyholder/Employer _____ *Thomson Reuters* _____

Claimant
Ira Fried

Part I. Personal Profile Evaluation (Please complete this form to the best of your ability. If you need additional space, please attach additional pages. Sign and date the form and promptly return it in the self-addressed envelope enclosed.)

1 . Please describe your most current medical condition or conditions (including the specific limitations or restrictions that they place on your ability to work). *Parkinson's and peripheral neuropathy. I get extreme fatigue from the Parkinson's ... the pain and tingling in my feet make it ... to visit or concentrate for more than an hour or two at a time.*

Has there been a change in your condition in the last 18 months? [ ] No [X] Yes If "Yes," please describe the specific change or changes. *The pain and tingling in my feet are new and seem to be getting worse on almost a weekly basis ... I need to spend at least a couple hours in bed each day ...*

2. Please list all of the types of activities that you do during the course of a typical day. What do you specifically do from the time you arise in the morning until you retire at night? Do you require assistance with any of your daily activities?
[X] No [ ] Yes If "Yes," describe: *I do most of the same activities I have always done. ... I read, send emails, talk to people on the phone, drive, etc. but I now am limited in how long I can do these activities. For example I can ...*

3. Please provide the following information about the condition causing your disability. Next to any Activity of Daily Living (ADL), please place the number shown next to the statement that most accurately reflects your ability/inability to perform each of them: 1 = I can perform this activity independently; 2 = I can perform this activity with the use of equipment or adaptive devices; 3 = I cannot perform this activity.

(1) Dress   (1) Voluntary bladder and bowel control or ability to maintain a reasonable level of personal hygiene
(1) Toilet   (1) Feed yourself with food that has been prepared and made available to you.
(1) Bathe (tub, shower, or sponge)   (1) Transfer from Bed to Chair

If you indicated 3 for any of the above activities, please describe the impairment and restrictions to your functionality that preclude you from performing the activity. *I can dress and bathe independently, but it can be very difficult and takes much longer than it used to.*

What is your Height: 6'1"   Weight: 195

Have you suffered a severe Cognitive Impairment that renders you unable to perform common tasks, such as using the phone, money management or medication management? [X] No [ ] Yes If "Yes," describe:

4. What kinds of hobbies or social/community activities did you engage in prior to your Disability? *running, hiking, playing catch with a baseball & or softball, bicycling, board games, volunteer work ... for dental ... organization*

Have you continued to engage in any of these activities since you became Disabled and/or do you presently continue with any of these activities? [ ] No [X] Yes If "Yes," please list the hobbies or social/community activities and how often you participate in them. *The only one of my physical activities I can still do is bicycling, doing so ... while I do ... exercise but I often cannot do so, due to foot pain. I still play board games occasionally. I spend on average about 10 to 15 hours per week doing ... volunteer activities ... mostly from home.*

5. Do you own a personal computer? [ ] No [X] Yes If "Yes," please provide the following information:

What types of programs are you proficient in? [X] Word [X] Excel [ ] Other _____

Do you have an e-mail address? [ ] No [X] Yes _____

Do you have your own web-site? [X] No [ ] Yes _____

See also attached

The questionnaire form I am required to fill out every 18 months—a difficult task for someone with Parkinson's Disease (my typewritten responses are reproduced on the following pages)

Claimant Questionnaire March 2011 responses

Question 1.

Please describe your most current medical condition or conditions (including the specific limitations that they place on your ability to work.

Parkinson's and peripheral neuropathy. I get extreme fatigue from the Parkinson's and the pain and tingling in my feet make it hard to work or concentrate for more than an hour or two at a time.

Has there been a change in your condition in the last 18 months?

Yes. The pain and tingling in my feet are new and seem to be getting worse on almost a weekly basis. I now need to spend at least a couple hours in bed every day due to the discomfort in my feet.

Question 2.

Please list all of the types of activities you do during the course of a typical day. What do you specifically do from the time you arise in the morning until you retire at night? Do you require assistance with any of your daily activities?

I do most of the same activities I have always done: walk, read, send emails, talk to people on the phone, drive, etc. But I now am limited in how long I can do these activities. For example, I can no longer sit at a desk for more than an hour or two at a time or for 3 or 4 hours in an entire day.

Question 3.

Please provide the following information about the condition causing your disability. Next to any Activity of Daily Living (ADL) please place the number shown next to the statement that most accurately reflects your ability/ inability to perform each of them: 1=I can perform this activity independently; 2=I can perform this activity with the use of equipment of adaptive devices; 3=I cannot perform this activity.

(1) Dress
(1) Toilet
(1) Bathe

(1) Voluntary bladder and bowel control or ability to maintain a reasonable level of personal hygiene

(1) Feed yourself with food that has been prepared and made available to you

(1) Transfer from Bed to Chair

I can dress and bathe independently, but it can be very difficult and takes me longer than it used to.

Height: 6'1" Weight: 195

Have you suffered a severe cognitive impairment that renders you unable to perform common tasks, such as using the phone, money management, or medication management?

No.

Question 4.

What kinds of hobbies or social/community activities did you engage in prior to your disability?

Running, hiking, playing catch with a baseball or football, bicycling, board games, volunteer work for charitable organizations.

Have you continued to engage in any of these activities since you became Disabled and/or do you presently continue with any of these activities? If "Yes," please list the hobbies or social/community activities and how often you participate in them.

The only one of my physical activities I can still do is bicycling. During cold weather, I use a stationary bike but I often cannot do so due to foot pain. I still play board games occasionally. I spend an average of 10-12 hours per week volunteering for charitable organizations, mostly from home.

Question 5.

Do you own a personal computer? If "Yes," please provide the following information:

Yes.

What types of programs are you proficient in?

Word and Excel.

Do you have an e-mail address?

Yes.

Do you have your own web-site?

No.

Addendum to Claimant Questionnaire—
Personal Profile Evaluation for Ira Fried

I have tried to answer the questions in your Personal Profile Evaluation by describing to the best of my ability, within the space provided, how I do on an average or typical day. But the reality is that there is no average or typical day. As I have come to understand is the norm for Parkinson's sufferers, I have my "on" times and my "off" times. During my "on" times my functioning is close to that of a healthy person: I am able to perform all of the activities of daily living; I am able to sit at a desk and work and I am able to walk short distances, all with moderate difficulty. During my "off" times I experience extreme fatigue and pain and/or tingling in my feet, which makes it extremely difficult for me to perform any of the activities of daily living, impossible for me to sit at a desk and do anything productive and difficult to concentrate on any one thing for more than a few minutes. During my "off" times, walking even a few feet is a challenging and painful experience.

I have both "on" times and "off" times every day. My physicians are trying to help me minimize the "off" times through medication, but even on my best days I am "off" for at least two to three hours. And on my bad days, I can be "off" for most of the day. I have a general idea of when the "off" periods are likely to start, based on the timing of my medications, but the length and intensity of my "off" periods is unpredictable, making it difficult for me to plan for when I can do anything productive.

The physician's statement provides detailed documentation of my medical condition as of 3/8/2011

Fax Server   3/7/2011 11:42:51 AM PAGE   2/004. Fax Server
------ ----.-- ---. Signed on 03/08/2011 7:37:38 AM

PATIENT: Ira Fried
DATE OF BIRTH: ... .
DATE: 03/03/2011 8:30 AM
VISIT TYPE: Return Visit

I had the opportunity of seeing Ira Fried in follow-up today for Parkinsons disease, Peripheral neuropathy,

Reason(s) for visit

Parkinsons disease, Peripheral neuropathy

Onset was 8 years ago. The problem occurs intermittently. Recently symptoms have not changed. Severity level is moderate. The patient exhibits idiopathic parkinsons disease. Context includes medication side effect. Tremor location(s) include the right upper extremity. They are described as resting tremors, dyskinesias. Medication side effects include tired/sedation, and of dose wearing off and peak dose dyskinesia. Aggravating factors include medication side effects. Relieving factors include medication and current med(s) have inadequately controlled symptoms. Associated symptoms include gait difficulty and h/o REM sleep behavior disorder. Symptoms interfere with work. Symptoms do not interfere with driving or ADL's. Mr. Fried has Parkinsons disease and peripheral neuropathy-possibly hereditary neuropathy. He has pain from his neuropathy that has not responded to Gabapentin 1500mg tid. He notes cramping pain in the toes that seem to relate to possible wearing off of Sinemet. He is does not wish to continue Comtan. Acupuncture has not helped with pain. He is interested in Big and Loud therapy after our discussion. I am suggesting a PD manual-Every Victory Counts. He can no longer work at any job secondary to pain, fatigue, concentration issues, and inability to sit for more than 1-2 hours at a time. He is on high dose Parkinsons medications without adequate benefit of symptom relief.

peripheral neuropathy

Onset was 2 year(s) ago and it was gradual. Duration is intermittent. Severity level is moderate. Location of pain and numbness is foot bilateral. The problem occurs constantly. Gait is characterized as unsteady. Symptom is aggravated by wearing off of meds. Relieving factors include medication (Neurontin not very effective) and no relief with acupuncture. Associated symptoms include nocturnal paresthesias, paresthesias, restlessness, tingling and cramping pain.

Allergies
No known allergies.
Medications

Brand	Dose	Description
Citalopram Hbr	20 Mg	take 1 tablet (20MG) by oral route every day
Clonazepam	0.5 Mg	take 1 tablet (0.5MG) by ORAL route every bedtime as needed
Comtan and levodopa	200 Mg	take 1 tablet (200MG) by oral route 4 times every day in combination with carbidopa

Ditropan XI	10 Mg	take 1 tablet (10MG) by oral route 2 times every day
Gabapentin	600 Mg	Take 2 pills three times a day
Requip	4 Mg	take 1 tablet (4MG) by oral route 3 times every day
Sinemet 25-100	25mg-100mg	take 2 tablet by ORAL route 4 times every day
Sinemet Cr	50mg-200mg	take 1 tablet by ORAL route every bedtime
Sinemet Cr	25mg-100mg	TAKE 1 TABLET DAILY FOR A WEEK THEN INCREASE BY 1 TABLET EACH

WEEK UP TO 1 TABLET FIVE TIMES DAILY 4 HOURS APART

Vital Signs

Enc. Date	Hgt	Wgt	Pulse	Sys.	Dias	Position	Temp	BMI
03/03/2011			68	112	64	standing		
03/03/2011			64	120	64	sitting		

Physical Exam
Neurological Single System Exam
Constitutional
The patient is in no distress.

Cardiovascular
No carotid bruit.
Heart rate and rhythm are regular. There was no murmur.

Musculoskeletal
Gait is impaired with dragging of the right foot, decreased arm swing. No freezing of gait or problems with turns. Mildly unsteady. Negative retropulsion with pull test. Normal muscle strength and bulk in all four extremities. Mild increased muscle tone/rigidity in the Right arm. Mild dyskinesias noted on exam. No resting tremors. Romberg's sign negative.

Psychiatric
The patient is alert and oriented x 3. Recent and remote memory are intact. Normal attention span and concentration. Normal spontaneous language and comprehension. Fund of knowledge is normal.

Neurologic
CN II - Pupils are equal, round and reactive to light and visual fields are intact. CN III, IV, VI - Extraocular movements full. CN V - No facial numbness to light touch. CN VII - No facial muscle weakness. CN VIII - Hearing intact to finger r.b. CN IX, X - Speech is clear. Palate moves in midline. CN XI - Shoulder shrug intact. CN XII - Tongue protrudes in midline. Test of coordination revealed normal finger to nose, and normal heel to shin. Finger taps, Hand rivmts slightly decreased on the right. Foot taps slightly decreased on the right-amplitude and speed.

Plan Summary
Appointments / Test Ordered

Plan Details	Comments	Date
Follow-Up Visit	Visit duration: 45 Minutes	03/24/2011
Referral	Refer patient to: physical therapy-Big and Loud therapy	

Assessment and Plan
Paralysis agitans (332.0)
Starting next week I will initiate a transition from Comtan to Sinemet CR 25/100 to be taken every 4 hours with regular Sinemet 25/250 totalling 5 doses per day. He will remain on Requip 4mg tid. We will try Big and Loud therapy. I suggested that he buy a PD manual online for informational purposes. I will see him back in 3 weeks to continue his medication changes. He will call if there are any problems. I wonder if some of his pain is related to end of dose wearing off as he describes cramping possibly dystonic pain in his toe/foot at the end of dose.

Neuropathy, idiopathic peripheral NEC (356.8)
This is painful for him. Neurontin (gabapentin) 1600mg tid has not been very effective and is causing side effects. Starting tomorrow, we will make the direct transition to Lyrica 100mg tid to see if this is more effective. He will call with problems. He will take this instead of Gabapentin. Repeat EMG could be considered after we make the changes to further delineate the cause or presence of neuropathy.

Extremities Pain (729.5)
Likely from neuropathy and from end of dose wearing off from his Parkinsons disease medications. We will make the changes above to see if we can give him further relief of his symptoms and I will see him back in 3 weeks.

Adverse Drug Effect (995.20)
Side effects on medications including high dose Gabapentin and dopaminergic agents. We will get him off of Gabapentin and make changes in other medications to try and help these problems.

Depression (311)
This is being managed by his psychiatrist Dr. Bruce Gimball with Celexa and counseling. He has REM behavior sleep disorder and is on clonazepam for that issue. Trazodone may be a possible option for depression and sleep after we make the above changes.

He is quite disabled by all of these issues impairing his ability to hold any type of employment. His pain, concentration, fatigue, and inability to sit for any period of time is quite difficult for him. I would be willing to fill out paperwork for disability if he so chooses.

Thank you for allowing me to participate in the care of your patient. If you have any questions or concerns, please do not hesitate to contact me.

Sincerely,

The medical decisions made by the nurse practitioner are consistent with our patient care practices. [. . . . .] MD was present in the office and available for consultation during this visit.

Document generated by: [. . . . .] z 03/03/2011 11:31 AM

CC Providers:

5

CHAPTER 18
DENIAL

Denial can be a funny thing. It is the first of the five stages of grief that Elizabeth Kubler-Ross says we need to go through to learn to live with a loss. In her writings, Kubler-Ross usually refers to the loss of a loved one. But the five stages can apply to any significant loss, including the loss of the ability to do something one loves—in my case, running. The path to acceptance—learning to live with one's loss—includes anger, negotiation, bargaining, and depression. Kubler-Ross describes denial as the stage in which "the world becomes meaningless and overwhelming." She also says that "denial is nature's way of letting in only as much as we can handle." Getting past denial and moving on to anger is a necessary part of the healing process.

Sometimes I find a small helping of denial can be helpful. I know I will have on and off periods every day and on my worst days the neuropathy pain I feel during my off periods might incapacitate me for several hours at a time. But I wake up each morning not thinking about the pain I experienced the day before or worrying about the pain I might feel during the day about to begin. I don't deliberately try to deny the pain. It just doesn't rise to the level of conscious thought. Instead my mind is filled with the places I need to go and the things I need to do that day.

I charge into each day blissfully unaware I may encounter an obstacle that could prevent me from doing everything I set out to do.

I rarely think about my long-term prognosis with Parkinson's and peripheral neuropathy. I just assume I will cope, no matter what happens. I know my condition will continue to deteriorate. But I keep my thoughts of it locked up in a cabinet right next to the cabinet that holds my painful childhood memories.

Perhaps one reason—and maybe the main reason—I feel so little anger about my illnesses is that I am stuck in denial. My natural inclination is to deny the reality of each milestone in the progression of my illnesses until the milestone moves into my past. Then I skip over anger, negotiation, bargaining, and depression and move right on to acceptance. By not dwelling on what I have lost and refusing to look forward at what I might become, I am able to focus on the present and live a full and productive life. In other words, denial helps me to be resilient.

This way of thinking is more than just a clever mental trick. It requires a considerable amount of practice. Several friends with whom I have shared these thoughts have likened it to Zen Buddhism—I live in the moment, unconstrained by past disappointments and fear of the future.

I think the Cognitive Behavioral Therapy (CBT) I learned years ago may also have helped. Predicated on the premise that our thoughts, both conscious and subconscious, determine our moods, CBT teaches us to replace our automatic negative thoughts with rational positive thinking. With enough practice, it is possible to eliminate much of the automatic negative thinking that leads to feelings of hopelessness and depression.

When I realized I could no longer do my job at Thomson Reuters, my automatic negative thinking went something like this: *Work and running gave meaning to my life and now I can no longer do either. I don't have any hobbies to keep me busy and the few friends I have are busy working all day. I don't know how I will spend my time. Soon, I will no longer have friends. My life as a productive human being has ended. My illnesses have sentenced me to a life of lonely misery. Poor me!*

But then my rational thought process took over. I rejected the notion that I could not find anything meaningful to do and started a Web search for volunteer opportunities. I accepted that I could no longer run and moved on to other types of workouts. I questioned the inevitability of no longer having friends. Casting off negative thoughts in this way led me from despair to something approaching a Zen-like state of acceptance.

Refusing to look forward at what I might become and not dwelling on what I have lost may be akin to resilience, but is not a silver bullet. Like most good things in life, too much of it can lead to some unintended negative consequences. I liken this way of thinking to sitting in the back of a car and looking through the rear window as someone else drives. As the car rolls forward I see new milestones of my illnesses' progression enter my past. They are easy to accept because I can see everything that has led up to them: *Look! There goes running drifting off into my past.*

Keeping my gaze on the past makes it easy to accept new limitations as they slowly but inevitably come into view. I take comfort in my ability to accept them so easily. Sometimes, though, I feel the need to take a more active role in coping with my illnesses. I need to get into the driver's seat. I can still look at the rear-view mirror, but I also need to face head-on some of the limitations my illnesses will soon impose. I need to fight back instead of passively accepting their inevitability.

One morning in spring 2011, I awoke from a vivid dream. The dream took place on a college campus. It started with a heated argument with a man I did not know. Next, I wanted to go for a run—indoors, because it was pouring outside. I looked all over campus for a place to run until finally I found a fitness center. I tried to go in, but a woman guarding the entrance told me I lacked the required authorization. I asked her if she could please make an exception for me, pleading, "I just want to run on the track. Nobody is using it now, so can I please go in?"

My plea failed to move her. She reiterated, "No, you cannot go in without a pass."

But as some people left the fitness center, the woman allowed several others to enter without a pass. Someone explained that the fitness center allowed people without a pass to enter so long as someone on their way out vouched for them. I saw the man with whom I had argued earlier leaving the fitness center and asked him if he would vouch for me. He said no and admonished the woman at the entrance to be extra vigilant and not to let me in.

Then the woman's supervisor appeared. I tried to plead my case to her but she also was unmoved. Outraged, I threatened to get a lawyer and file a lawsuit against the fitness center, but the supervisor refused to budge. Then the manager of the fitness center entered my dream. She had overheard the argument; concerned I might go through with my threat, she intervened. She went to a kiosk next to the entrance and typed my name. A few moments later she told me that, since my record indicated I had done very well in college and was highly qualified to run, she would let me in.

Next, I was on the track, running hard. For a moment I had the track to myself but then another runner appeared right in front of me. I tried to stay on his shoulder, just like I used to do during the track workouts with The Group. It felt great to be working out on a track again.

As I left the fitness center I noticed the manager admonishing the woman at the entrance and her supervisor to be more careful about who they denied entry. But then, as I passed the manager, she told me she had allowed me into the fitness center as a one-time exception. I started contemplating the argument I would use the next time I encountered her. Then I awoke.

This dream sent me a clear message—I had given up on running too easily. If I fought back maybe I could run again. It would not be easy, but I needed to at least try. Perhaps a Freudian psychiatrist would have discerned other meanings from my dream, but the possibility of running again resonated so strongly with me that it crowded out any other possible interpretations.

A few days later Joy and I went for a walk around our neighborhood. I had not run for over two years, but feeling especially energetic that morning, I wondered out loud whether I could run the 100 feet or so between two mail boxes. I also wondered what it would mean if I could. Joy, demonstrating her penchant for finding practical answers to my deep philosophical quandaries, suggested I stop talking about it and just try. So I did.

I ran between the two mailboxes with surprising ease. Elated, I tried running twice the distance. Again, I did it without difficulty. Shocked, but ecstatic about my new-found ability, I decided to test myself by running a 3.2-mile loop around the neighborhood. Joy cautioned me to try a shorter distance first but, recalling I used to run five miles on my *easy* days, I ignored her advice.

I ran comfortably at a slow but steady pace for the first two miles. Then my legs started to hurt. But I pushed on, determined to prove to myself, and the world, that I could do the entire run. By the 2.5-mile mark, my legs felt as if they were filled with sand. Each step became a new experience in pain. But the pain just made me more determined to keep going. By the time I got to within a quarter mile of my house, I no longer could claim to be running—my slightly bent-over posture and swinging arms belied the fact that I now kept at least one foot firmly planted on the ground at all times as I inched forward. Finally, I turned the last corner and saw my house come into view about a hundred yards away. I no longer felt any pain; it had been replaced by fatigue more intense than anything I had ever felt before. Each step forward now required a monumental effort. Finally, after expending every ounce of energy and will power I had, I touched the mailbox and collapsed onto the grass. After lying there for several minutes, I got up and shuffled to my house.

The next day I felt worse than I had the day after any

of my marathons, by several orders of magnitude. It took me the next full week to recover. But I was elated—I had reclaimed running from the list of things I could no longer do.

I settled on a 1.4-mile loop, which I ran three to four times a month during the warmer months through 2012. These runs thoroughly exhausted me, but I felt the same sense of satisfaction after finishing that I used to feel after a strong twenty-mile run.

My 3.2-mile run may have been a little extreme, but I think it is important to push myself from time to time to test the boundaries between what I can and cannot do. This principle applies as well to intellectual endeavors and social situations. I have taken on some challenging assignments for the three charitable organizations on whose boards I served—for example, taking the lead role in developing strategic plans for each of these organizations. That and my writing have helped to keep my mind sharp—or at least sharper than it would otherwise be. And I avoid a natural tendency to hide within myself by actively seeking opportunities to socialize with both old friends and new acquaintances. In today's vernacular I look for ways to get out of my comfort zone. And in so doing I am able to slow the rate at which my illnesses cause it to shrink.

A Final Word on Resilience

I have stated that resilience has been key to "handling my illnesses well." I have also said that, while some people may be born with a greater disposition for resilience than others, it is a skill that can be learned. I believe the practice I gained during a difficult childhood has helped give me the resilience I have needed to cope with Parkinson's and peripheral neuropathy. I also believe that some of the choices I have made since receiving my diagnoses have made it easier for me to be resilient. Most important has been my decision to volunteer by serving on the boards of charitable non-profits. In the early years of my illnesses, I joined three such organizations: Summer Camp Scholarships, which sends low income children to summer camp; Partners in Personal Assistance, which provides non-medical, in-home care for people with disabilities; and Michigan Ability Partners, which provides housing and support services for otherwise homeless people with disabilities.

When I was actively volunteering, I spent only a few hours each week helping these organizations, but the work I did reassures me I am still capable of living a productive life. I often feel I accomplished more in the few hours I devoted to these organizations each week than I did in the fifty-plus hours I used to spend at my paying jobs.

On a more practical level, my volunteer work gave me a reason to get out of the house and/or do something each day. Had I not joined the boards of these organizations, I might have found something else. But I also can imagine myself having fallen into a vicious circle of getting depressed at having nothing worthwhile to do and then turning in to myself rather than looking for something productive to do, and so on.

I would be remiss not to acknowledge I have some advantages that make it easier for me to be resilient. For one, I have a good health insurance plan, which gives me access to world-class medical care. Second, I am lucky I do not have to worry much about money. Most important though, is the unflagging support Joy gives me. It goes far beyond reassuring me that she will be there for me as my condition worsens. In her work as a home care speech therapist, she frequently sees patients whose lives have been changed by a serious illness—for example, people who have recently suffered strokes. She has a genius for connecting with these people and recommending small changes that make a huge difference in their lives. She does the same for me.

Joy is a confidante with whom I can share my deepest fears about my illnesses. But at the same time she manages to strike a perfect balance helping me when I need it while not allowing me to become dependent on her. She usually recognizes my limitations well before I notice them and am willing to accept them. Hers is the voice that awakens me from my denial when it becomes counterproductive. More times than I can count I have had an epiphany regarding how I can compensate for the limitations my illnesses impose only to realize a day or two later that for the last several weeks Joy had been telling me what I just discovered.

· · · · · · · · ·

I needed more than a heavy dose of resilience when I learned in March 2011 I had a large mass on my kidney. The growth turned out to be benign, but when it was first discovered, I did not know this. I needed a belief system to help me understand why, after having exercised daily, not having smoked or abused alcohol and having eaten a healthy diet since the age of fourteen, I had just been diagnosed with my third serious disease. Since my early teens,

I had thought often about God's existence and how to live a moral life. I fondly remember the countless hours I spent debating these issues with my friends in college. But still, I did not have a set of beliefs I could articulate and call upon to help me cope with this new life-threatening disease. Then lightning struck.

CHAPTER 19
THIS I BELIEVE

During one of our long "meaning of life" discussions, Jim told me about his "This I Believe" essay, explaining that *This I Believe* was a program on National Public Radio which encouraged its listeners to submit a 500-word essay that identified their core beliefs. Submissions accepted by a review board were added to a database and one essay was selected for broadcast each time the show aired. Jim said the exercise of summing up his core beliefs in a 500-word essay had helped him figure out what was most important to him in life. He suggested I also try writing one of these essays. After reading his, I was intrigued, but I didn't think I would ever get around to writing one myself.

Then, about four months later, I was doing a power walk while listening to my favorite Dylan album, *Blood on the Tracks*. About a week had passed since my urologist had told me the tests she'd ordered confirmed the mass on my kidney was most likely cancer and she would have to remove the kidney. I wasn't consciously thinking about my medical condition. I was nearing the end of my walk when I heard the following lines from "Buckets of Rain," the last song on the album:

Life is sad,

Life is a bust.

All you can do is do what you must;

You do what you must do and you do it well.

These words hit me like a lightning bolt! They summed up the missing piece of my spiritual belief system—what I need to do to live a meaningful life—more clearly than any words I could have composed myself. I knew immediately I would have to write down my thoughts in my own "This I Believe" essay. And as Joy can attest, I was obsessed with this essay until I finally completed it four days later.

To me, the first two lines of Dylan's verse mean you cannot always control what happens in life; sometimes you are lucky enough to have good things happen, sometimes not. In my case, with the kidney cancer diagnosis heaped on top of my peripheral neuropathy and Parkinson's, life was pretty bad at the moment. But Dylan doesn't dwell on how sad life can be; he just states it as a fact and accepts it. And I knew that is what I should do, too.

Accepting that life can be bad does not mean giving up. Quite the opposite: to me it means trying that much harder to do what it takes to make a positive difference, for myself and for others, during whatever time I have left on this earth. It is not merely important to do these things; it is essential. I *must* do these things if I am to live a meaningful life. That is the meaning I take from "All you can do is do what you must."

The last line, "You do what you must do and you do it well," means it is not even enough to do what is essential. That is only half the battle. It is equally important to do it well. After all, if you don't do it well, what's the point of doing it at all?

Dylan doesn't say exactly what it is you must do. Each person needs to figure that out for him or herself. But for me, that was the easy part. I knew I needed to finish the job of raising my two boys. I knew I needed to keep my mind and body active for as long as I could. I knew I needed to give something back to my community by volunteering. And now, I knew I needed to tell my story.

Doing it well, however, does not mean simply doing a good job at the three or four things I consider most important in life. It means much more than that. It also means showing respect for the people I meet regardless of their station in life. It means being thankful for the gifts I have received. It means being willing to extend a helping hand to someone in need. And it means acting with a sense of humor and humility but also a sense of dignity. Simply put, it means being a decent human being.

I realize I do not always do it well. Being human, I often fall short. But I believe knowing what I must do and how I must act to do it well provides the moral compass I need to live a worthwhile life.

The rest of my belief system did not come so easily. I have been thinking about this topic on and off since I first started to doubt what I was being taught in Hebrew School when I was twelve years old. My beliefs are the culmination of what I learned in school; ideas I have picked up from books, articles, and discussions with friends; and my experience dealing with adversity.

My core belief, upon which the rest of my beliefs rest, is that the most important questions religions address are unanswerable by rational thought. Does God exist? If so, is God a sentient being who knows and cares about each of us? How does God want us to behave? I believe answering these questions requires an act of faith. As a result, no one set of beliefs or religion is more correct than any other. And most important, it is impossible to prove any one group of people or set of religious beliefs is more favored in the eyes of God than any other.

My beliefs help me make sense of the world and cope with the adversity I face with my illnesses. They are an important part of who I am. I share them with some reluctance because I fear they may offend some readers who have strong beliefs that are different from mine. But I feel that not to share them would be to not tell my whole story. I am not trying to convert anyone to my way of thinking. But I hope that just maybe, by sharing my beliefs, I might help others make sense of the world in a way that helps them cope better. So with those caveats, an explanation of the rest of my belief system follows.

The three questions I ask above provide a useful framework for me to explain my beliefs. I had thought often about the first question, "Does God exist?" and had been frustrated by my inability to come up with a logical argument that would answer the question one way or the other. The question seemed unanswerable, but I could not prove that either. Then, at about four o'clock one morning during finals week of my sophomore year in college, I had an epiphany. I had been working since early evening on an essay on Kant for a class in Western philosophy when suddenly, it came to me. I finally understood Kant's logic for his assertion that some things, including the existence of God, are unknowable. His conclusion—that we need to take a leap of faith to accept God's existence—made complete sense to me. Kant had validated a belief I had held for a long time but could not articulate. I have long since forgotten the details of Kant's logic—I recently re-read my essay and found even my summary of his logic to be almost impenetrable. But his central point, that belief in God requires an act of faith, remains a core belief of mine.

Armed with the knowledge that all I needed to do was take a leap of faith, I leaped. But I didn't make it to the side of faith. I just couldn't summon the faith that God exists. So I became an atheist.

But I still had some niggling doubts. And these doubts grew stronger over time. I had no answer to the "intelligent design" assertion that, while science may help to explain what *is*, we need God to explain *why*. With the rapid advances in genetics, science explains more about us every day. But no matter how much science explains, I am still left with the question, *why?* I finally realized my belief that there is no God was every bit as much a leap of faith as the belief that God exists.

After my kidney cancer scare I once again looked for an answer to this question. I talked about it with friends. I did some reading. And after a considerable amount of thought I took another leap. This time I landed in the chasm between belief and disbelief. I am not sure whether God exists. I am now an agnostic.

The second question—"Is God a sentient being who knows and cares about each of us?"—is easier for me to answer. I just cannot see how it is plausible that such a God exists. I have another friend, Jas, with whom I also sometimes get into "meaning of life" discussions. Several years ago, I shared my beliefs with him and Jas replied with a story. Long before we met, he saw a dime on the sidewalk and bent down to pick it up. While he bent down, a drunk driver's car careened off another car and flew airborne, inches over Jas' head. Had he not bent down to pick up the dime, he would have been killed instantly. After telling this story, Jas opined there must be some cosmic force that led him to bend down at precisely the right moment to save his life.

Jas' story is hardly the first I have heard of someone avoiding a catastrophe or experiencing a life-changing event that seemingly can be explained only by divine intervention. But I have never seen proof of divine intervention. And I believe I never will because divine intervention is not provable—it is a matter of faith. I believe it is equally impossible, however, to prove that divine intervention does *not* exist. For that reason, I consider Jas' belief to be every bit as valid as my own, even though I may disagree with it.

I would like to believe in a cosmic force that looks out for us, but I have too many questions. Just a few days before Jas told his story, I heard a piece on the news about how, during Hurricane Sandy, a man died when a tree fell on his house, crushing him instantly. The neighborhood had been evacuated and the man should not have been in the house. Still, his death appears to have been a freak accident. I cannot help asking, did some cosmic force make this accident happen or choose not to prevent it from happening? Why would God choose to save Jas' life and let this man die? And what of the hundred-plus other people who died in the storm? Is God really an arbitrary and capricious cosmic force that sometimes acts beneficently, sometimes malevolently, and other times not at all? These questions lead me to take the leap of faith that even if God, the creator, exists; God, the all-knowing, all-powerful, loving being does not.

I realize this notion of God raises an equally difficult question. If God did not cause Jas to bend down to pick up the dime at just the right moment and is not responsible for the other seemingly miraculous stories we have all heard, how then do we explain them?

The answer, or more accurately, *my* answer, to this question eluded me until about a year and a half before I started to write this memoir. Then, spurred on by a book, an extremely unlikely coincidence, and a number of long discussions with Jim, I developed this part of my belief system.

Fooled by Randomness, by Nassim Taleb, addresses the errors we make when we think about luck. The book focuses mainly on financial markets but most of the lessons in the book apply equally to life in general. The two most important lessons for me were: 1) We tend to underestimate the role luck plays when we are successful and overestimate the role that luck plays when we are unsuccessful; and 2) We routinely underestimate the probability of seemingly highly improbable events.

A few weeks after I finished reading *Fooled by Randomness,* Joy, the boys, and I went to Sanibel Island for the week of school winter vacation. Not long after we settled in to our rental condo, I received a strange email from Jim. He wanted to know where we were because his daughter had just told him she was positive she had seen Sam just a few minutes earlier. Jim and I quickly established that we were both on Sanibel Island and were staying at the same condo development. That seemed like a pretty remarkable coincidence to me. Then, a couple of hours later, I went out to the balcony of my unit. Much to my surprise, I heard Jim's voice. He was in the unit next to ours.

Jim and I were both early risers and the rest of our families were not, so we decided to go to a coffee shop for breakfast each morning. And, as is often the case with Jim and me when we have enough time to talk, our conversations veered to "the meaning of life." During this week I developed and refined my belief that we live in a probabilistic universe. If we had perfect information, I reasoned, we could determine the probability of every significant event that has happened in our lives. And now, buttressed by the lessons I learned from *Fooled by Randomness*, I knew many of the events that seemed highly improbable to me when they happened may have been much more likely than I had originally thought.

Take, for example, the coincidence of Jim and me ending up in condo units next door to each other on Sanibel Island. First, it must be noted that the odds were actual pretty high we would choose the same week to go there, as our children had the same week off for winter break. We had both been to Sanibel Island and planned to return. Still, it was quite a coincidence that we ended up at the same development in units next door to each other. But as Nassim Taleb explains, random encounters with friends or relatives are not as improbable as we think. "It is just that we should not be testing for the odds of having an encounter with one specific person, in a specific location at a specific time." Rather, we should be testing for any encounter, with any person we know, in any place we visit. And the latter probability is several orders of magnitude higher than the former.

A similar explanation applies for the man who died during Hurricane Sandy and Jas' near-death experience. The odds may have been low for that individual to die from a tree falling on his house and crushing him. But every time a natural disaster is reported in the news, it seems we learn of someone dying in a similarly tragic manner. And while Jas' survival from his experience may seem incredibly lucky when viewed as an isolated event, the odds go up considerably when we consider all the other times he went for a walk and nothing memorable happened.

To be clear, I believe probability theory offers an *explanation* but is not a *cause* for the events that make up our lives. Luck certainly plays a role in our lives. But we also make our own luck by the actions we take and the decisions we make. Yes, I had the good fortune to receive an excellent education and have a genetic make-up that includes a strong aptitude for math. But I also made decisions along the way that gave me more options and increased the probability of positive outcomes. I believe in free will. And I believe that the more we take control of our lives by exercising our free will, the easier it becomes to do so in the future. This practice makes us better able to respond in a positive, self-determined way when life takes an unexpected turn for the worse.

Thinking about the world in this probabilistic way helps me to cope with my illnesses. I do not dwell on why I had this misfortune because I know there is no answer. I know I just had bad luck. I am able to accept this reality and move on with my life. And when I find myself asking "Why me?" I remind myself that in so many other ways, I have had exceptionally good luck.

Finally, I do not believe in heaven and hell and I do not believe that we have a soul that lives on after we die. But I do believe we live on in the memories people have of us and in the impact we have had on their lives. Over the years, I have had numerous dreams about my father. In many of these dreams he helped me to deal with a difficult situation. In this way, he still lives within me. I hope the people who read this memoir discover some truths or think about some things in new ways that are helpful to them. I especially hope my boys, and some day, their children, will read it, so I remain alive in their memories and the impact I have had on their lives lasts long after I have died.

Following are responses to questions in the 9/9/13 Claimant Question-naire and 9/13/13 Physician's Statement filled out by my neurologist.

By the time of the 9/9/13 application for continuation of disability benefits, my handwriting had deteriorated so much it was largely illegible. The typewritten questionnaire responses shown here were a joint effort by Joy and me.

Once again, the physician's statement provided by my neurologist shows the status of my medical condition as of 9/13/13.

Claimant Questionnnaire September 2013 responses

I have tried to answer the questions in your Personal Profile Evaluation by describing to the best of my ability how I do on an average or typical day. But the reality is that there is no average or typical day. Like most people with Parkinson's, I have my "on" times and my "off" times. At this point, my "on" times are short-lived and are often accompanied by dyskinesia. That, combined with the need to stay off my feet as much as possible due to the neuropathy pain makes it difficult to do normal household chores. I can sit at my desk and pay bills, write e-mails, etc., but usually for no more than an hour at a time. During my "off" times, I experience extreme fatigue and pain and/or tingling in my feet, which makes it extremely difficult for me to perform many of the activities of daily living, impossible for me to sit at a desk and do anything productive and difficult to concentrate on any one thing for more than a few minutes. During my "off" times, walking even a few feet is extremely painful.

I have both "on" times and "off" times every day. My physicians are trying to help me minimize the "off" times through medication, but even on my best days I am "off" for at least two to three hours. And on my bad days, I can be "off" for most of the day. I have a general idea of when the "off" periods are likely to start, based on the timing of my medications, but the length and intensity of my "off" periods is unpredictable, making it difficult for me to plan for when I can do anything productive.

Below are my answers to questions 1 through 4. I have answered the rest of your questions on the form.

Question 1.

Please describe your most current medical condition or conditions (including the specific limitations that they place on your ability to work.

I continue to suffer from Parkinson's and peripheral neuropathy (PN). These are both progressive diseases, which means my symptoms will gradually get worse over time. My Parkinson's symptoms that now most affect my ability to work are fatigue, difficulty concentrating on a task for more than about an hour at a time, diminished ability to multi-task, and poor balance (which has led to several recent falls). Also, the dyskinesia from my Parkinson's medications has forced me to limit my driving to short distances. My handwriting is almost illegible at times due to the tremors in my right hand and the dyskinesia.

The pain I experience from PN has become considerably worse over the last 18 months despite my physicians' best efforts to control it with medicines. I feel constant pain in my feet, which requires me to keep off of my feet as much as possible. I also experience episodes of intense pain that often are debilitating–all I can do is lie in bed until the pain subsides. There is no average or typical day. I usually have at least one episode a day lasting two to three hours. But the episodes can be as short as 45 minutes to as long as six hours.

I was diagnosed with lymphoma in April, 2013, but my lymphoma is indolent and has not yet had an impact on my daily life.

Question 2.

Please list all of the types of activities you do during the course of a typical day. What do you specifically do from the time you arise in the morning until you retire at night? Do you require assistance with any of your daily activities?

I continue to do most of the same activities I have always done: walk, read, send emails, talk on the phone, drive, etc. But I have become more limited in my ability to do these activities. For example, I now use a cane to walk and I have to limit the time I spend on my feet as much as possible. I also avoid driving for more than 20 minutes at a time and when I am experiencing a neuropathy pain episode, avoid driving at all. Whenever someone with a driver's license is in my car with me, I ask them to do the driving. I no longer drive at all at night. I have had to quit my volunteer work for non-profit charitable organizations because I no longer have the energy to attend meetings and keep up with emails. It takes me longer to write emails due to my dyskinesia and I have had to reduce the amount of time I spend doing volunteer work for charities, due to fatigue, my PN foot pain and my diminished ability to concentrate. I rely on my wife to get things for me when I am experiencing a PN pain episode

Question 3.

Please provide the following information about the condition causing your disability. Next to any Activity of Daily Living (ADL) please place the number shown next to the statement that most accurately reflects your ability/ inability to perform each of them.

I can still perform all of the listed tasks independently, when I am not having a neuropathy pain episode. I occasionally have to rely on my wife to close a button. I eat slowly because tremors and dyskinesia often cause food to fall off my fork before I can put it in my mouth.

I have experienced additional cognitive impairment over the last 18 months. It has not rendered me unable to perform the common tasks listed.

Question 4.

What kinds of hobbies or social/community activities did you engage in prior to your disability?

Activities I did before my disability included working, running, hiking, playing catch, bicycling, going to movies and concerts, and volunteer work for charitable organizations. When I am "off" I cannot do any of these activities. When I am "on" and my PN pain is mild I can do power walks and ride my bike. But I am now able to do these activities only two or three times a week. I still occasionally go to movies and concerts, but I have to avoid staying out past 9:00 due to the PN pain. I am no longer able to volunteer for charitable organizations. For bladder control I take meds, but also need to wear Guards for Men.

Please fax the completed form to:

ATTENDING PHYSICIAN'S STATEMENT OF CONTINUED DISABILITY

To be completed by the Employee

Patient Name: Ira Fred   Date of Birth: ured ID Number:

Patient Address: (Street, City, State & Zip Code):   Ann Arbor, MI, 480?

Email Address:

Personal Cell Telephone Number: (   )   Alternate Telephone Number: (   )

May we have your authorization to leave confidential medical and benefit information on your personal cell phone? ☑Yes ☐No

I hereby authorize release of information on this form by the below named physician for the purpose of claim processing.

Signed: Ira Fred   Date: 9/9/13

To be completed by the Attending Physician - Use current information from your patient's most recent office visit or examination to complete this form. (The patient is responsible for the completion of this form without expense to the Company.)

DIAGNOSIS

Primary diagnosis: PARKINSON'S DISEASE   ICD-9 Code: 332.0

Secondary diagnoses: NEUROPATHY   ICD-9 Code(s): 355.9

Current Subjective Symptoms: SLOWNESS, FATIGUE, PAIN

Current Physical Examination findings: BRADYKINESIA, RIGIDITY, ABNORMAL GAIT

Current Blood Pressure: 117/65   Height: 1.667 m Weight: 90.99 kg Weight Loss or Gain?

Current Pertinent Test Results (Not previously reported; List all results, or enclose test result reports):

Test: Date: Results:

Test: Date: Results:

Current Medications, Dosage, and Frequency (indicate any changes): AMANTADINE 100mg BID, AMITRIPTYLINE 25mg QHS, SINEMET CR 25/100 5x/DAY, SINEMET 25/250 5x/DAY, COMTAN 200mg 5X/DAY, LYRICA 300mg BID

TREATMENT PLAN

Current Treatment Plan: CONTINUE MEDICATIONS

What is the Frequency / Duration of Treatment? EVERY 6 MONTHS Dates of Treatment: 8/8/12

First Office Visit for this condition: 12/9/08   Last Office Visit: 8/13/13   Next Scheduled Office Visit: 2/9/13

Has Surgery been performed since last report: ☐Yes ☒No If "Yes," on what Date(s):

Procedure(s):   CPT Code(s):

Was patient hospitalized since last report? ☐Yes ☒No If "Yes," Hospital name and phone Number:

Admission date: Discharge date:

Has patient been referred to other physicians? ☐Yes ☒No If "Yes," Date of Referral(s):

Referral Physician Name   Phone Number: (   )   Specialty:

Referral Physician Name   Phone Number: (   )   Specialty:

LC-7137-6 [LTD FF]   Page 1 of 2   09/2012

Fried, 2PA (pg 2)

FUNCTIONAL CAPABILITIES

Please complete the applicable portion of this section based on your most recent clinical assessment.
In a general workplace environment the patient is able to:

	Sit	Stand	Walk
Number of hours at a time	0	0	0
Total hours / day	0	0	0

Please circle / check the frequency that the patient can perform the following activities:

R = Right L = Left B = Bilateral		Never	Occasionally (1-33%)	Frequently (34-67%)	No Restriction
Lift / carry 1 to 10 lbs.		R L (B)	R L B	R L B	R L B
Lift / carry 11 to 20 lbs.		R L (B)	R L B	R L B	R L B
Lift / carry 21 to 50 lbs.		R L (B)	R L B	R L B	R L B
Lift / carry 51 to 100 lbs.		R L (B)	R L B	R L B	R L B
Lift / carry over 100 lbs.		R L (B)	R L B	R L B	R L B
Bending at waist		✓			
Kneeling / Crouching		✓			
Driving		✓			
Reaching only (not load-bearing)	Above shoulder	R L (B)	R L B	R L B	R L B
	At waist / desk level	R L B	R L B	R L (B)	R L B
	Below waist / desk level	R L (B)	R L B	R L B	R L B
Fingering / handling		R L (B)	R L B	R L B	R L B

Is the patient's vision impaired? ☐ Yes [✓] No   If "Yes", please describe the extent of the impairment. _____

Best corrected vision: R _____   L _____

Does the patient have a psychiatric / cognitive impairment? ☐ Yes [✓] No   If "Yes," please describe the extent of the impairment and its etiology: _____

Expected duration of any current restriction(s) or limitation(s) listed above: LIFETIME _____

Do you believe the patient is competent to endorse checks and direct the use of the proceeds? [✓] Yes ☐ No

PHYSICIAN INFORMATION

Provider's Name _____	Telephone Number: _____
Degree: M.D. Specialty: NEUROLOGY	Fax Number: _____
License Number: _____	Social Security Number or EIN Number: _____
Street Address: _____	City: ANN ARBOR State: MI Zip Code: 48109
Signature: _____	Date signed: 9/13/13

LC-7137-6 (LTD FS)   Page 2 of 2   09/2012

CHAPTER 20
THE LONG WAY HOME, PART I

I had looked forward to this trip for months. Jim and his wife, Sue, both business school professors at the University of Michigan, had decided to use their sabbatical year to take a trip around the world, meeting with colleagues along the way. Before embarking on the overseas portion of their trip they stopped for three months in Eugene, Oregon, where most of Sue's family lives. Needing a car for these three months, Jim drove his own out to Eugene. He planned to drive back to Ann Arbor at the end of the trip in July 2013. He asked me if I would like to join him.

Jim explained he would pick me up in Eugene or Portland—my choice—and we would have eleven days to get from there to Ann Arbor. I could choose whatever route I wanted so long as Jim and his car made it back to Ann Arbor on time.

I imagined myself as Dean Moriarty, the hero in Jack Kerouac's iconic *On the Road*, crisscrossing the country with his friends. Like Dean and his companions, Jim and I cared more about the journey than the destination. Yes, I chose a route that included some popular tourist sites, like Yellowstone National Park, Mount Rushmore, and the Badlands. But the spirit of travel was the same as Dean's. We would be out on the open road, exploring whatever captured our interest along the way. I expected nothing less than a journey of self-discovery, with my best friend Jim prodding me along. I could hardly wait.

· · · · · · · · ·

My adventure began with a non-stop flight from Detroit to Portland. I had found an inexpensive one-way, first-class ticket, which enabled me to travel in comfort. I arrived at my hotel late Friday morning feeling rested and looking forward to spending the next two days exploring Portland on my own.

The trip came at a time when I badly needed some time away from home. A couple of months earlier, Partners in Personal Assistance (PPA) had failed a government audit that accounted for forty percent of its revenue. A week later, Lena, PPA's Executive Director and a long-time leader in the movement that encouraged people with disabilities to live self-directed lives and gave them the resources they needed to do so, announced she planned to take an indefinite leave of absence to have major heart surgery. A few weeks later she died of complications from the surgery. I discovered at Lena's standing-room only memorial service that she was a friend and hero to hundreds of others in the community, as well.

A few of us on the board formed an ad-hoc emergency committee to determine how best to respond to the challenges we faced. My three-to-five-hour a week commitment had become nearly a full-time job. I attended strategy meetings, reviewed proposed policies, drafted position statements, and so on. Most evenings I spent an hour or more on the phone coaching Jody, the board chairperson. I had become physically, mentally, and emotionally exhausted. I told Jody I needed a break from PPA and vowed to myself that during the trip I would keep my PPA work to a bare minimum.

The tension gradually lifted from my shoulders as I wandered around Portland on Friday and Saturday. But on Sunday morning I checked my emails and saw I had received an urgent request to participate in a meeting that afternoon. The purpose was to discuss our strategy for dealing with the audit. I knew I should keep my promise to myself to take some time off from PPA. But I couldn't help it—PPA needed me and I couldn't let the organization down. I arranged to call in to the meeting.

Within the first ten minutes of the call, I could feel all the tension come back again, pressing on my shoulders harder than it had before I boarded my flight in Detroit. The other board members had decided that during a meeting with the auditor scheduled for Tuesday, they would make a major concession I thought we neither had to nor should make. I thought that, with some education, the auditors would realize their demand was unreasonable and they would back down. Frustrated and concerned about PPA's future, I tried to argue against making the concession. But I got nowhere.

After the call ended I went for a long walk to try to calm myself down and get PPA off my mind. I felt much better an hour later when I returned to my room. I took a long hot shower, finished packing and then alternated between reading the book I had brought along and dozing off. Shortly after three I left my room, checked out, and sat in the lobby waiting for Jim to arrive. I passed the-time playing a game on my cell phone—anything to avoid thinking about PPA.

Jim finally arrived a few minutes before four. Six feet tall, with a shaved head and a thin athletic build, he was clad in a worn T-shirt, too-short shorts, running shoes, and white socks. He exuded energy but looked rattled as he bounded out of his car and strode over to greet me.

Jim's appearance belied his status and accomplishments. A professor at the University of Michigan's business school, he has won just about every honor available to someone in his profession. A few months before he went on sabbatical he turned down an offer to become Dean of the business school at one of the top universities in the country.

The back seat and trunk of Jim's lime-green Honda CRV were crammed with boxes of books, clothes, and various other items he needed to take back with him to Ann Arbor. But he somehow found a place for my bags, while leaving plenty of room for me to stretch my legs and recline my seat if necessary during a neuropathy attack. We stopped for a quick bite to eat and then started on our journey eastward. First stop: Boise, Idaho.

It didn't take long for us to strike up a conversation. Jim, always affable, but normally calm and relaxed, was as frazzled as I had ever seen him. Two weeks earlier, he had returned to Eugene from his year-long whirlwind tour around the world. The next day, without taking time to adjust to the nine-hour time zone change from France, he launched into a flurry of activity that culminated with meeting me at my hotel. Among other things, Jim had driven back and forth to San Francisco twice, made multiple trips to the local airport and arranged for the transport of his and Sue's things back to Ann Arbor. But the main event had been his niece's wedding and the several parties that followed. Jim's niece had asked him to preside over the wedding ceremony as minister—a great honor. Jim recounted in great detail how he had written the sermon, how well it had been received by everyone in attendance and, most poignantly, how proud of him it had made his daughter.

I was genuinely interested in and impressed with the process Jim had gone through to write the sermon—internet research, consultations with ministers he knew, multiple drafts, and so on. I listened actively, frequently asking questions. But I did feel a tinge of regret that my relationship with my two boys was not nearly as close as was Jim's with his three daughters. At the time, both Alan, twenty years old, and Sam, almost seventeen, were struggling with the transition from adolescence to adulthood and neither seemed interested in my offers to help.

Occasionally, Jim interrupted himself or I interrupted him to comment on the scenery. I had not expected the landscape to change so quickly and dramatically as we passed from lush mountains to the desert-like high plains. Most remarkable to me, though, were the wind farms. They stretched on for upwards of twenty miles, with hundreds of huge wind turbines dotting the ridges of the hills on either side of us. I wondered how much of the area's energy needs the wind farms provided. By then, PPA was the furthest thing from my mind.

After about four hours on the road Jim told me he was starting to feel tired. He said he planned to stop at the next exit to take a catnap of maybe twenty to thirty minutes. I offered to take over driving for a while, but Jim demurred, saying he felt it would be safer if he did all the driving. I insisted, pointing out the sparse traffic and how straight and flat the road had become. Jim relented and I drove for about an hour without incident. While I drove and Jim slept, my thoughts unintentionally returned to PPA. I could not stop perseverating about it. I felt I had to do something to steer PPA in the right direction.

Jim took over the driving again and about forty-five minutes later, just past ten, we saw a sign listing the Boise exits. Caught up in our conversation, I hadn't kept track of the time. *Wow, I just survived a six-hour drive without any neuropathy pain,* I thought to myself. *But I hope staying up this late won't have negative repercussions tomorrow.*

For the last couple of years I'd rarely stayed out later than nine or nine-thirty. When Joy and I went out for dinner and a movie, we went to a late afternoon movie first and then to dinner. I wasn't afraid I would turn into a pumpkin at the stroke of nine-thirty, but by then the combination of neuropathy pain and fatigue usually made active participation in conversation difficult. Most days I started getting ready for bed at about nine. I then spent close to an hour to wind down and get in bed, ready to go to sleep. An on-and-off insomniac, I found if I didn't give myself enough time to unwind before going to bed I had trouble falling asleep. My Parkinson's and neuropathy made everything take that much longer, especially when I experienced a particularly bad neuropathy attack.

Jim and I had talked openly about potential conflicts and contingencies long before the trip. We agreed to split the cost of gas, take turns paying for meals, and pay for our own rooms. We also talked about where Jim could drop me off to fly home if the long hours sitting in the car proved to be too much for me. The only issue that required much discussion was when we would start and end the day. Jim preferred to get off to a late start after spending time in the morning to go for a run, read the paper, and check emails. Then he liked to drive until eleven or twelve at night. I preferred to get off to an early start and end the day by nine or nine-thirty. We agreed to split the difference.

Jim got off the highway at the first Boise exit after seeing a sign for a Holiday Inn Express. We checked in and asked where we could find a place to eat. Nothing was open at that time—10:15 on a Sunday night—but fortunately the hotel had leftovers from its Sunday buffet. By the time we finished eating and I got into my room, it was close to eleven. I should have gotten ready to go to sleep. But first I had to save PPA. So before doing anything else I took my laptop out of its bag, connected it to the hotel's Wi-Fi and started banging away at an email to PPA's board. I couldn't help myself. I needed to convince the board not to make the concession to the auditor we had discussed on Sunday morning.

As I typed away I intermittently looked at the alarm clock on the night table beside my bed. I knew if did not get enough sleep I could practically count on having bad neuropathy the next day, but even as I saw the clock go past twelve, then twelve-thirty, and then one a.m., I kept working on my email. I needed to make a logical and forceful argument to convince the board to reverse course. I needed my email to be perfect. I re-wrote a couple of paragraphs several times until I was satisfied they were just right.

I finished writing the email at one-thirty, and finally got to bed at two. *Tomorrow might be a little rough*, I thought to myself, *but I have done what I needed to do.*

I woke up later that morning, at eight, and before doing anything else checked my phone for replies to my message. Nothing. I would check my email at least a dozen more times that day; I received not a single reply.

I took the pills I had laid out before going to bed, got dressed, and went down to the lobby for breakfast. Jim had just finished when I arrived. He needed some time to reply to some emails, so we agreed to meet in the lobby, ready to check out, at ten.

My feet hurt, but no more than usual for the first hour or so each morning after taking my meds. A couple of bagels, a banana, and three cups of coffee later I was fully awake and ready to start the day. I was glad to have the extra time, though. That would give the meds time to fully seep in before I had to lug my bags from my room to the elevator and from there to Jim's car. It took no small effort for me to move the suitcases, even with rollers. Among other things, I had packed a couple of ten-pound weights—I used them for a workout I had devised in which I laid on my back and alternated between bicycle kicks and quick bench-pressing repetitions.

With our next destination, Jackson Hole, Wyoming, only five-and-a-half hours away, we decided to take a few minutes to check out the University of Idaho campus. We had strolled around for twenty minutes or so when Jim noticed a sign for the Idaho History Museum. Not particularly interested in Idaho history and wanting to get my workout in while I had the chance, I asked Jim if he minded if I did a power walk while he explored the museum. He didn't.

I walked for forty minutes and despite the near ninety-degree heat, had a good workout. The lack of sleep didn't seem to have had much effect on me. Jim, meanwhile, had satisfied his curiosity after about ten minutes in the museum and spent the next half hour waiting for me. A little annoyed, he said we needed to figure out a better schedule for our workouts. But he also said he had chatted with the guard at the museum, who told him about a quintessentially Boise hamburger joint that featured over forty flavors of French fries.

I had sworn off fried foods some years earlier, but readily agreed to go to the place the guard had recommended for lunch. Like Jim, I wanted to get a little taste of the local culture in each place where we stopped. The restaurant did not disappoint. More hamburger shack than restaurant, the place bustled with activity. I searched for and luckily found an open table while Jim waited on line to place our orders. I normally ate something light and healthy for lunch, but the aroma of the burgers frying on the griddle and the youthful, energetic atmosphere of the place were too hard to resist.

Hungry from having just worked out, I greedily devoured the hamburger and mountain of sweet potato fries the cook had heaped on my plate. I washed it down with a forty-ounce cup of Diet Coke. After eating we lingered for a few minutes to buy T-shirts and chat with the owners. Then we got back into the car and continued on our journey.

We reached Jackson Hole, a picture postcard of a town

known mainly as a ski resort, at about five. To Jim's and my surprise the town was full of hikers, bicyclists, rock climbers, and all other manner of tourist-athletes. We were lucky to find a motel with vacancies for $175 a night. We explored downtown Jackson Hole until about six. Then, both of us still full from the delicious but greasy lunch, we headed to one of the ski resorts. That was where my troubles began.

As we approached the base of the mountain I started to feel discomfort in my stomach. By the time we reached the parking lot the situation had become urgent. Jim dropped me off so I could rush to the men's room while he parked the car. False alarm. I had suffered from constipation on and off for at least twenty years, but this was worse than any other time I could remember. I gave up after a few minutes and looked for Jim.

I found him in the souvenir shop. Jim enjoyed taking the time to look for just the right gift for each person on his list. By contrast, the only thing I liked less than shopping was root canal surgery. When Jim picked me up at my hotel in Portland he had given me a T-shirt he found in Budapest that said "Life is Good: Enjoy the Ride," a message that perfectly evoked the creed I had tried to live by since learning of my illnesses. I wore that T-shirt proudly.

Jim said he wanted to spend another half hour or so there and then drive to another ski resort on the other side of town that had a mountain-top restaurant. He had read in a travel guide that the views from the restaurant were spectacular, especially at sunset. And the resort gave free gondola rides up and down the mountain to patrons of the restaurant.

Not wanting to get back to our motel too late, I suggested we stay where we were. This resort we were at did not have a mountain-top restaurant and it charged twenty-four dollars per person for the gondola ride, but I reasoned that the views from the top of this mountain would be every bit as stunning as the views from the mountain-top restaurant and we could get back to our motel at least an hour earlier than if we went to the other place. I offered to pay for both of our tickets and Jim reluctantly agreed. After another unsuccessful trip to the bathroom, I bought the tickets. Soon enough we were on our way up the mountain.

I had long considered mountains to be the most beautiful places on earth and these were no exception. We could see for miles in every direction. We stayed there for over an hour. I finished my exercise for the day by walking down a gentle ski slope for about fifteen minutes and then walking back as fast as I could. Meanwhile, Jim talked to a couple he had befriended on the way up. I wanted to join them after my walk, but first I had to rush to the bathroom again. Again, no luck.

By the time we got back on the gondola my stomach discomfort overwhelmed the adrenalin rush I got from my walk. I just wanted to get back to our motel. I thought it couldn't get much worse—but, as I would soon realize, this was just a warm-up for the main event.

As we started down the mountain I started to feel tingling in my toes—a telltale sign a neuropathy attack was on its way. I couldn't predict how long an episode would last or how badly it would hurt. It might be relatively mild and last for as little as forty-five minutes. But it also might be debilitating and last for several hours. I took some comfort in knowing I had taken all my meds at the right time—something I failed to do about once a week, on average. But I had forgotten how little sleep I had gotten the previous night. Lack of sleep almost always made my neuropathy pain worse.

The tingling grew more intense by the minute. I had joined Jim in a conversation with his new friends, but by the time we got halfway down the mountain, all I could think about was how much my feet hurt. I didn't notice my stomach pain anymore.

We got off the gondola and Jim, noticing my discomfort for the first time, asked me if I would like him to get the car while I waited. I gratefully accepted the offer. A few minutes later he pulled up about twenty feet from where I had sat down on some grass. I struggled to get on my feet and shuffled to the car, moving maybe six inches with each step. Then, with what felt like herculean effort, I got into the car. By this time I also felt feverish, which often happened during my worst neuropathy episodes.

The moment I got into the car, Jim's and my relationship changed. No longer a couple of old buddies on a road trip, we had morphed into brothers with a close but dysfunctional relationship. Jim became the caring but often insufferable older brother and I became the striving but inept younger brother. Although imperceptible at first, this change soon permeated every interaction we had through the end of the trip.

I tried to mitigate the pain by concentrating on breathing, a technique I learned during a meditation class I had taken the previous summer. Jim, unaware of how bad the neuropathy pain had become, razzed me about my constipation. "Why were you running to the bathroom every fifteen minutes?" he asked. I told him and he said laughing, "I hope you don't make a mess in my car."

Not wanting to engage in discussion, especially about my bodily functions, I said, "I can't guarantee it," then resumed my breathing exercise.

Jim waited a few seconds before asking, "How long has it been since you have taken a shit, anyway?"

I wanted to change the topic, or better yet, stop talking altogether. But I knew Jim wouldn't let up. "About two weeks," I lied, not wanting to admit it had really been closer to four weeks.

"Geez, you ought to do something about that."

I knew Jim was right, but I desperately wanted to end the conversation; the neuropathy pain had become almost unbearable. Finally, we arrived at our motel. I was in no condition to carry my bags, so I accepted Jim's offer to bring them to my room for me. He told me to give him a call when I was ready to go out to dinner.

It took about an hour for my neuropathy pain to diminish to the point where I could walk again. I called Jim at about eight and we went to a restaurant the motel manager had recommended to Jim. The place could best be described as an over-priced, touristy, cowboy steak house. There were several large rooms, the walls of each covered with photos depicting the Wild West. The restaurant was full and the noise deafening. The hostess and waitresses, including ours, were all young and beautiful. Jim chatted up our waitress each time she came to our table. I tried to join in a few times, but it seemed that each time I thought of something witty to say the conversation had already moved on to the next topic.

By the time we left the restaurant, at about nine-thirty, my neuropathy pain had become a distant memory. I still felt bloated from the constipation, but no longer had the urge to run to the bathroom every fifteen minutes. I was back to my old self.

After laying out clothes for the next day I checked my phone for emails one last time. Jody had responded. She wrote that she agreed with me but didn't know what to do because the rest of the PPA board wanted to go in the opposite direction. After reading Jody's email I concluded that I needed to take one more shot at convincing the PPA board to change direction. *If I can get an email out tonight, I* hoped, *maybe someone else on the board will read it before the nine o'clock meeting with the auditor and together with Jody might convince the others not to make the concession we had discussed on Sunday.* I promised myself I wouldn't stay up late writing a long detailed email as I had the night before. I finished a few minutes before eleven and went to sleep at about midnight.

Jim and I had agreed before we went to our rooms that we would pack, check out of the motel, and be ready to go at nine-thirty the next morning. We had a big day ahead of us. We planned to drive to Yellowstone National Park, about an hour from Jackson Hole to the west entrance, and spend most of the day in the park. Then we would head to Cody, Wyoming, where we would spend the night. Cody was an hour-and-a-half drive from the east entrance of the park and was the only town for miles around. Not getting off to an early start meant either not having much time in Yellowstone or getting into Cody late at night.

The next morning, I woke up at about eight. Despite staying up late again, I felt well-rested and easily handled a milder-than-normal morning neuropathy episode. I got dressed and walked to a bakery a couple of blocks away, where I bought a large cup of coffee and a muffin for breakfast. After eating I went back to the motel, checked out, and returned to my room to finish packing. I looked forward to seeing Yellowstone. But as I was about to leave the room, my stomach started rumbling again. I made another unsuccessful trip to the bathroom after which I felt more bloated than ever. That made me nervous. I thought about Jim's concern about my going just two weeks without a bowel movement and Joy once telling me that a bowel obstruction can be very serious, even deadly. Once we left Yellowstone, the nearest doctor might be several hours away. *What a shitty way to go*, I thought to myself in a moment of dark humor. I decided to play it safe. I called my primary care doctor to ask her whether I needed any medical attention. I reached a nurse and told her the truth about my situation. She told me I needed to go to the emergency room right away.

When I told Jim he acted not the least bit annoyed. I thought that, had our roles been reversed, I would not have been nearly as calm and understanding as Jim. Jim packed my belongings in his car and we headed toward St. John's Medical Center. When we arrived at the emergency room, Jim told me apologetically that he wasn't going to stay with me at the hospital. Instead, he planned to go back to town and try to find a coffee shop with Wi-Fi so he could catch up on his emails and get some work done. He said he hoped I did not feel abandoned. I had exactly the opposite reaction. Surprised that Jim felt responsible for watching over me and embarrassed by the whole situation, I replied, "Not a problem. I'll just call you on your cell when they finish with me." I felt I owed Jim the apology.

In retrospect, I think Jim was more concerned about me than I was for myself. I still saw myself as an athlete, the guy who used to run twenty miles every Sunday. True, I now regularly used a cane. And true, I now could barely finish the 1.4-mile course in my neighborhood that I used to use as a warm-up for my hard twelve-mile runs. But I could still run—occasionally. And I could still get by on my own. In my mind, Parkinson's and peripheral neuropathy hadn't diminished me in the least. I graciously accepted help when offered—like when strangers held doors open for me or when Jim put my bags in my room—but I never asked for it. Why would Jim even think I needed him to wait for me in the emergency room? I was, after all, fully capable of taking care of myself. Wasn't I?

I began to understand that Jim saw me in a completely different light than I saw myself. For example, I wondered why Jim had been so reluctant to let me drive while he took a nap as we approached Boise. Now the answer was abundantly clear: he didn't feel safe with me behind the wheel. I learned later that, before the trip, Joy had urged him not to let me drive. When Jim finally did let me drive, he insisted I use cruise control. I hadn't realized I had been pumping the gas pedal, causing the car to repeatedly surge forward and then slow down. Jim also had seen me lose my balance and nearly fall countless times. And he had seen me shuffle to the car, barely able to move, the day before. Jim saw me as someone who needed help and a watchful eye.

I walked into the emergency room and was relieved to see that, unlike many of the rural hospitals I had toured as a consultant, this place was modern and spotlessly clean. I signed in and joined the other five or six people in the room who sat waiting for the nurse in charge to call their names. Not more than ten minutes after I arrived she barked out my name. I got up and followed her to the imaging room, where a technician took several x-rays of me. Then the nurse led me to an exam room and told me to wait there for the emergency room doctor. I obeyed. Much sooner than I had expected, the doctor knocked on the door and came in. He showed me the x-ray so I could see for myself what I already knew: my colon was stretched full of stool. He said he would try to clean me out first with an enema, and if that didn't work, move on to a more invasive treatment.

I had hoped to be treated by a kindly, elderly, female nurse. Instead, I was greeted by Mitch, a fortyish-year-old man who stood about 5'10"and must have weighed at least 200 pounds, all of it muscle. He announced he would be the nurse administering the enema for me. Twenty painful minutes later, after what had to have been the biggest shit I had ever taken, I could shit no more, despite Mitch's words of encouragement. Mitch said, "Okay. We're done." I did not hear him say, "For now."

The enema seemed to have done its job. Relieved to be finished with the ordeal, I reached for my clothes only to hear Mitch say, "Slow down there, fella. We're just getting started." Three more enemas and about two hours later I was done for real. I got dressed and waited for the doctor to check me out. He gave me what I thought was a prescription, but turned out to be the name of an over-the-counter drink. He advised me to drink it the next time I got blocked up. I headed back toward the emergency room at about two p.m., feeling better than I had when I entered, but still not quite right.

I walked through the nearly-empty emergency room toward the exit thinking I would sit on one of the benches just outside and soak up some sun while I waited for Jim to pick me up. But before I reached the exit the receptionist stopped me and said, "I think somebody is waiting for you." I had walked right by Jim without seeing him.

We got in the car and I apologized profusely for the delay my visit to the hospital had caused. Jim insisted it was really no problem; he needed the time to catch up on things and had a productive morning. Jim laid out the plan for the rest of the day. He said it was too late to drive to Yellowstone, so we should stay in Jackson Hole for another night. He suggested we get some lunch, find a motel—which turned out to be even more expensive than the motel we had stayed at the night before—and then go to a grocery store, where I could find my medicine and he could get some things he needed.

Jim, apparently unaware of my embarrassment, asked a stream of questions about my ordeal. And, having caused us to waste a day and spend close to $200 for another night in Jackson Hole, I felt obliged to answer at least some of them. By the time we reached the grocery store, he probably knew as much about my bowel movements as my parents had when I was an infant. At the grocery store Jim insisted on helping me find just the right type of adult diapers, which I would wear for the rest of the trip just in case. On the way out of the store I fumbled my bags and dropped the drink the emergency room physician had recommended. The bottle exploded on impact with the floor. By now, feeling like a complete doofus, I implored Jim not to go back inside to get another bottle. Thankfully, he didn't. We went back to the motel, where I rested for the remainder of the afternoon.

CHAPTER 21
THE LONG WAY HOME, PART II

The next morning we got off to an early start and headed toward Yellowstone. Not long after leaving Jackson Hole we came across one of the most awesome sights I had ever seen. In front of us and to our right the terrain was as flat as a table top. But to our left, and what seemed like just a few miles away, the flat Great Plains abruptly ended. Instead there rose a huge mountain range. It looked almost as if someone had carefully placed the mountains on the edge of the Plains. Jim stopped the car so we could get a better look. He took a picture of me with the mountains in the background. Then he asked me to do the same for him.

For as long as I can remember I have been bad at anything requiring even the smallest amount of aptitude with spatial relationships. Knowing this, I have studiously avoided any task that requires this skill. When Joy and I moved our old TV from the family room to our bedroom, I had no problem figuring out where to plug in all the cords to make the TV work with the cable box, DVD player, and Netflix box. But I needed Joy's direction to get the TV through the door to our room. Whenever we bought something that required assembly, Joy put it together. I had owned my smart phone for over a year and had yet to use the camera.

Jim explained to me that anyone could take a picture with his phone camera. I just needed to center him in the frame and click. It was that simple. I followed Jim's instructions but none of the pictures I took came out right. I failed to align most of them correctly, giving Jim a haircut or cutting him off at the knees. For the rest, I put the entire frame at an angle, as if the world had tilted. On a number of occasions, Jim placed the camera in my hands at exactly the right spot and then scurried back to pose for the picture. All I had to do was hold the camera steady and click. These pictures came out no better than the others. Each time I tried to take a picture I demonstrated my incompetence again. After a few days of this Jim stopped asking me to take pictures. I should have stopped. But I was hell-bent on getting at least one picture right. Not until weeks after the trip did I realize that tremors and dyskinesia made it nearly impossible for me to hold my hand steady enough to take a decent picture.

We arrived at Yellowstone just in time to get good seats to see Old Faithful. I had seen it as a seven-year-old and had seen it on TV a number of times on nature shows. But still, it amazed me to see the steam spew out of the ground and shoot up a hundred feet or more into the sky at the appointed time.

As we explored more of the park it became apparent that Yellowstone had far more to offer than geysers and boiling pools of mud. The waterfalls, among the most spectacular I had ever seen, the herd of bison grazing in a meadow, and the acres of charred remains from the 1988 fire all were memorable to me.

All in all, it was a great day. I rated Yellowstone a close third to Yosemite and Lake Tahoe as the most beautiful places I had ever seen. With all the walking—including a

600-step walk down and back up to the viewing area for one of the waterfalls—I had gotten my daily exercise, and then some. My legs felt so tired, they hurt. But this was the good type of tired, like how I used to feel after my long Sunday runs. I had almost forgotten about my stomach problems and PPA. The other PPA board members, incidentally, were proven right some six months later. All my worrying had been for naught.

What I will remember best about our day in Yellowstone is an incident that could have happened almost anywhere. At about six, after having crammed as much sightseeing as we could into a one-day driving tour of Yellowstone, we were ready to head to our next stop: Cody, Wyoming. We had about a forty-five-minute drive along a winding, hilly road to reach the park exit before we would begin the hour-and-a-half or so drive to Cody. Jim, who once again had done all the driving, announced he was tired and pulled the car into a small gravel rest stop. He said he needed to take a catnap before continuing on. Despite my tired legs, I was wide awake. I offered to drive while Jim slept and he reluctantly agreed. As I settled into the driver's seat, Jim pulled out his pillow and rested his head against the passenger window. Then he yawned and, already half asleep, muttered through a wan smile, "Please don't get me killed."

A few seconds later I almost did just that. I looked back and, noticing I could see only about 200 feet behind me before the road curved downward and to the left, I gunned the engine. But for some reason the car moved haltingly, no more than about ten miles an hour. I should have looked back again, but for the next few moments I focused entirely on the car and my inability to make it accelerate. *Why won't the car move faster?* I asked myself in alarm as I pulled out of the rest stop and onto the shoulder of the road. Then, before I had time for another thought, a pick-up truck flew around the bend, missing us by no more than a foot. The truck had to be moving at close to sixty miles an hour. Had it hit us, we would have been seriously injured or killed.

Jim, hearing the truck whoosh by us, jolted upright just in time to see it hurtle past before it disappeared around the next turn. I pulled the car completely off the road and turned off the engine. After taking a moment to catch his breath, Jim asked if I had seen the truck almost hit us. I sheepishly answered that I had. Then Jim said several times, half to himself and half to me, "At least I'm awake now." I tried to apologize, but what can you say to someone after having almost killed him? To Jim's great credit, he uttered not a single word of recrimination. He didn't need to. I couldn't have possibly felt worse. Left unsaid but understood, I would not be permitted to go anywhere near the driver's seat for the rest of the trip.

· · · · · · · · ·

With the benefit of hindsight I can at least partially explain the sequence of events that led to our near-disaster. First, Jim put the parking brake on but did not tell me. I never used the parking brake when I drove my own car and had no reason to expect that Jim would use his. He had not used the parking brake when I took over driving on the first night of the trip. The brake had prevented the car from accelerating.

Second and more important was the impact Parkinson's had on my thought process during The Incident. One of the cognitive effects of Parkinson's is to make multitasking more difficult. Most people automatically think of several things in quick succession when they drive, usually without even realizing it. The thought process for someone without Parkinson's might have gone something like this: *Nothing on my left. Why won't the car accelerate?* Quick look to the left again. *Wow, that truck was moving fast. The car still won't accelerate. I can't be moving this slowly when I get on the road. Better stop and ask Jim what's wrong."* But with my Parkinson's, I got stuck on one thought: *Why won't the car accelerate?*

Parkinson's may help to explain what happened but it does not absolve me of responsibility for the near-accident. Upon recognizing I could not see very far to my left, where the cars on my side of the road were coming from, I should have reminded myself to take one last look before I started out. Better yet, I should have told Jim that the limited sight distance made me uncomfortable and asked him to drive to a safer place before I started driving.

. . . .

Jim drove the rest of the way and we reached Cody at about eight. As we stood in the motel office waiting to check in, Jim struck up a conversation with the hotel manager. I admired Jim for taking a personal interest in everybody he met, but I also wanted to get into my room. After about fifteen minutes of chatter, I literally and figuratively couldn't stand it anymore. I interrupted the conversation in mid-sentence, asking the manager to please check me in.

Startled and clearly annoyed with my poor manners, the manager silently took my credit card, motioned for me sign the registration, and gave me my room key. As had become our custom, Jim unloaded my bags from the car and placed them in my room. Jim and I agreed to meet for dinner in fifteen minutes. He went back to the office to get a restaurant recommendation while I rested.

We went to a steakhouse the manager had advised Jim had great food and was a favorite of the locals. The restaurant greatly exceeded my expectations. If there is such a thing as an authentic Western restaurant that ranchers go to on their big night out, this would be the place. The pictures on the wall were of regular people doing mundane ranching tasks, like herding cattle into their pens, milking the cows, and so on. There were no heroic pictures of the Wild West like at the restaurant in Jackson Hole. The menu entrees consisted of several cuts of steak and nothing else. In the middle of the restaurant, down a few steps, a live band played country music while people danced. Jim and I took our time savoring our steaks and soaking up the atmosphere. Jim, ever the extrovert, made no less effort to get to know our waitress here, an average-looking, forty-something mom, than he had the hottie at the restaurant in Jackson Hole. We did not get back to the motel until after ten—another late night.

The next morning Jim said he wanted to make up some time. He set as our goal Rapid City, South Dakota, a six-hour drive from Cody. A couple of months earlier, while planning the trip, we talked about Rapid City as the most logical place for me to stop and fly home if necessary. But ending the road trip prematurely never crossed my mind. Despite my misadventures, I had no intention of stopping until we reached Ann Arbor. For his part, Jim did not so much as hint that I should fly the rest of the way home.

. . . .

I looked forward to a long day on the road. I had asked Jim to critique the memoir chapter I'd written on my belief system and finally we would have plenty of time for him to give me his feedback.

I played a lot of pick-up basketball in college. The best games were when everyone took it seriously and gave their best effort. The rules were simple: just don't try to hurt anyone. Otherwise, no blood, no foul. I went all out during these games, as if my life depended on winning. But as soon as the game ended I no longer cared whether I had won or lost. I was happy for the opportunity to participate in a hard-fought contest. Win or lose, I always made a point to thank my opponents for the game.

Jim and I had argued about God and religion since we were roommates in graduate school. It was a kind of sport for us. Our discussions about God, religion, and beliefs were similar to those pick-up basketball games. I always look forward to them and Jim is one of the few people I can have them with. I never held anything back, nor did he.

As a business school professor, Jim was accustomed to reviewing scholarly articles in a highly rigorous and critical manner. Did the article recognize previous work on the same topic? Did it use sound methodology in coming to its conclusions? Were the findings interesting and meaningful? And so on.

My "This I Believe" chapter failed to measure up on all accounts. I had presented my ideas as entirely my own, as if no one before me had considered we live in a random universe without a caring, benevolent God. I hadn't explained in a logical manner how I reached my conclusions—they just came to me in a moment of insight. And worst of all, my conclusions were neither interesting nor meaningful. "So what if we live in a random universe where things happen for no good reason," Jim exclaimed. "What does that tell us about how to live our lives?"

I told Jim that my belief system included a set of moral principles—my interpretation of the stanza from Bob Dylan's "Buckets of Rain," which I'll repeat here:

Life is sad,

Life is a bust.

All you can do is do what you must

You do what you must do and you do it well.

I told Jim why these words were so important to me. I explained how in a flash of insight, my lifetime of thinking about God and morality—asking questions like how an all-knowing, caring God could exist in a world with so much suffering and randomness; why I won the three disease lottery; and how I can live a meaningful life despite my illnesses—coalesced into a belief system that answered these questions for me. I went on to say I was not trying to convert anyone to my beliefs. They helped me to make sense of the world and my place in it. And they helped me to deal with the adversity I faced. I told Jim

I thought that everyone needs to have something to believe in. For many people that "something" is a loving, caring God. For others it is a belief in human progress made possible by science and innovation. I reminded Jim my "This I Believe" chapter was not intended to be a scholarly article that should be subject to the rigors of peer review. I wrote it merely to explain, not to defend, what I believe.

My explanation did not move him. He wanted to know where my ethical beliefs came from. I responded "the Dylan song," my frustration growing.

But that answer only raised more questions for Jim. "What made you interpret the song that way?" Jim pressed on.

I had no answer. "What does it matter?" I asked, starting to feel a little defensive.

Then Jim dropped a bomb. "There must be something divine in you that gives you these moral principles," he argued. Now feeling more than just a little defensive, I felt the blood rush to my head in anger. I had not heard an argument like this since my college friend, Jim F, had told me that because I was an ethical person, I must believe in God, even though I didn't know it.

What arrogance, I recalled thinking. *How could he presume to know more about what I thought about God than I did myself?*

Back in the car, the other Jim took the argument a step further. He suggested it was I who was arrogant. I, after all, thought I could develop my own set of moral principles without the help of God. Jim suggested I show some humility by allowing for the presence of God in my life.

Perhaps sensing my anger, Jim deftly changed the subject. He asked me if I wanted to take a detour to see Devils Tower. Not until then had I bothered to notice the beauty of the Black Hills we had been meandering through for the last several hours. I happily said yes. I badly needed a break from our discussion and welcomed any opportunity to see an interesting natural sight. Devils Tower, a mound of dirt and basalt that rises straight up 1,267 feet above low, gently-rolling hills, is one of those phenomena in nature that seem too strange to be real. It looks like it was put there by aliens. Stephen Spielberg must have had the same reaction. In his movie, *Close Encounters of the Third Kind*, a small cadre of believers in world and universal peace gather at Devils Tower. There, they board an alien ship. For Jim and me, our time there was a welcome respite from our discussion about God, morality, and the meaning of life. We changed into our walking/running clothes, and Jim went for a run while I did a two-laps-around-the-tower speed walk. We arrived back at Jim's car forty minutes later, both of us refreshed from the exercise. A half hour later we were on the road again.

After a few minutes exchanging comments about the wonders of Devils Tower, Jim began talking about a problem that he had been working through with one of his daughters. Since the first night of the trip, he had talked about this issue as it had unfolded. He told me how he and his daughter had exchanged long emails and spent hours on the phone talking about the issue. He said he thought they had finally resolved it. Everything would be okay. I wondered at first in silence and then out loud why I did not have a similar relationship with Alan or Sam. I could barely get them to talk to me at all, much less rely on me for guidance on an issue of importance to them.

Jim then said, "The relationships Sue and I have with our daughters are the culmination of years of us demonstrating our love for them in many small moments. Haven't you and Joy also had countless small moments like that with Alan and Sam?"

Jim meant his question to be rhetorical, but feeling defensive and insecure, I took it as a challenge. Joy and I had been active, engaged parents with both of our boys from the moment they were born. When they were little, Joy and I had taken them to a museum or zoo almost every weekend. We rarely missed one of their soccer or baseball games. Joy and I had regularly checked in with them on their homework and offered assistance whenever they needed it. We had advocated for them at school on numerous occasions. Joy now frequently reminded me our boys would have to figure things out by themselves. But why? Why couldn't we help them figure things out now?

For one of the few times during the trip, Jim and I had run out of things to talk about. Thinking it might lighten our mood, I suggested we listen to one of my books on tape. Jim agreed and we listened to *The Emperor of All Maladies*, a history of the treatment of cancer. Two hours later we began to get bored with the book. Also, Jim was ready to give me more feedback on my belief system.

This time, Jim didn't critique my belief system so much as urge me to allow the divine into my life. He said he saw me as someone who is living a good moral life, but without a moral compass. He saw me struggling to make sense of the world. If I would just take away the barriers I have built to letting God into my life, I would find peace. He told me how he had found peace by letting God back into his life after years as a lapsed Catholic, and how several friends of his had done the same. I listened as he continued his appeal for the next few hours, at once gratified that he had taken such an interest in my spiritual well-being and annoyed that he felt he had to.

We finally started seeing signs announcing our imminent arrival in Rapid City, South Dakota. As Jim exited the highway and we started looking for a hotel, I felt the beginning of what I knew would be an intense neuropathy episode. My belief system did nothing to prevent these episodes. Would allowing God into my life make a difference? I doubted it.

While I focused on my breathing in an effort to control the pain, Jim found a comfortable hotel. After checking in, he loaded all my stuff onto a luggage cart. Fighting the neuropathy pain all the way, I barely made it to my room. When I got there the pain was too much for me to hold the door open while pushing the luggage cart through. I was stuck. I thought about calling Jim on my cell phone, but before I had a chance, I saw him come out of the elevator and run towards me. He pushed the luggage cart into my room, unloaded my belongings and took the cart back out. He told me to call him when I felt well enough to go out to dinner. I said okay, while secretly resenting him for the help he had just given me. Why couldn't I handle this situation by myself?

We had a long drive planned for the next day, with the Badlands the major sightseeing destination on our route. The Badlands had intrigued me for a long time, so I was looking forward to finally getting to see them. We got off to a late start and did not get to Badlands National Park until early evening. The landscape was even more bizarre than I expected. With the exception of the occasional tuft of grass, it looked like a moonscape. I could see how some conspiracy theorists might use it as evidence that the moon landings had never really happened. The park itself was tiny compared to Yellowstone but the desolate land surrounding the park stretched out as far as the eye could see. It would be miles before we reached the next hint of civilization, which meant it would be another late night. I recall thinking to myself that this would be a really lousy place to run out of gas—but not a concern for us, as Jim had filled the tank before he started out that morning. I was glad for the opportunity to see this strange and forbidding land.

It had been drizzling all morning and afternoon but shortly after we left the park the drizzle turned into a steady rain. The darkened sky cast a pall over the landscape, making it feel even bleaker than it had just a few minutes earlier. Each of us in his own world, we traveled in silence for the next hour or so. I do not recall who broke the silence, or who started the conversation, but we soon became engaged in a fierce debate about abortion, capital punishment, gay rights, decriminalization of drugs, and the like. I had partaken in frequent debates on these topics during college and had long considered them to be an important part of my college experience. But this time was different. Jim had launched into a full frontal assault I felt was directed not at the issues, but at me personally.

After what seemed like hours, I saw the first sign on the highway announcing the presence of some small towns not far off. Twenty minutes later the first signs for

Mitchell, South Dakota, appeared. Meanwhile, the rain came down harder. Jim increased the fury of his assault, as if egged on by the rain.

Refusing to give in, I tried to defend my positions. But then I started to feel a neuropathy episode come on. The pain, relatively mild at first, soon became as intense as any episode I had ever experienced. Jim, apparently unaware of my condition, pressed on. I tried to keep up my side of the argument, such as it was, but soon found communication of any kind nearly impossible. In my weakened state, Jim caught me in a contradiction. He cried out in victory, "You don't even know what you think." By then I was happy to surrender if it meant stopping the argument. Before I had a chance to do so, Jim noticed me writhing in pain. He graciously ended the argument saying, "Hey, I'm good at asking questions, but not so good at answering them."

When we arrived at the hotel, Jim had to check both of us in and then come back to the car to help me to my room. I could not have made it by myself. Jim muttered something about getting pizza for dinner while I crawled into bed. A half hour later Jim returned with the pizza. Feeling much better, I greedily ate more than my share. Then Jim left the room, I crawled back into bed, and went to sleep.

· · · · · · · · ·

The last night of the trip we stayed with our mutual friend from Northwestern, Don, and his wife JoAnne at their house in Madison, Wisconsin. It had been over ten years since we had seen each other at the 2003 Boston

Marathon. Jim parked the car and we walked toward the front door, where Don greeted us. We took a moment to look at each other, and said in unison, "You look…" None of us wanted to complete the sentence. Jim finally blurted out "older," ending the awkwardness. I can only imagine after Don saw me move how much more he must have thought I had changed. We exchanged pleasantries for a few minutes and then started talking about Don and JoAnne's kids.

A couple of hours later JoAnne arrived and we ate dinner. We had a great time reminiscing about the past. I went to bed at eleven—way past my normal bedtime— while Jim, Don, and JoAnne stayed up and continued talking. I woke up at six the next morning and went to the kitchen, where I found JoAnne. We started talking and within a few minutes the conversation turned to our children. JoAnne shared with me how challenging it had been at times raising hers. This conversation meant a lot to me. Knowing that child-rearing could be challenging, even for people like Don and JoAnne, restored my confidence—maybe I wasn't such a bad parent after all. And maybe Joy was right, too. Our boys will figure things out, but in their own time and in their own ways. Sometimes, as Dylan writes, all we can do is do what we must: let our kids know we love them and that, as long as we live, we will be there for them.

· · · · · · · · ·

I fell into a deep funk after arriving home. The trip had sapped me of my physical, mental, and emotional energy. I couldn't write for over three months. I tried several times

310

but each time I wrote maybe two or three lines, which I tried to edit, but ultimately deleted. I went to my writing group, where the leader and other members had consistently praised my work. This time I felt as though I was under attack. They said I had painted a picture of living with my illnesses that was just a little too easy. They were right. I had described an early stage of my illnesses, before they had begun to affect my life in a meaningful manner.

At first I blamed Jim. Why did I feel so much anger at him? I resented him for his energy, self-confidence, and plans for the future. I thought these things were no longer available to me. At times Jim angered me for being clueless about my condition. At other times he annoyed me for understanding my condition all too well. And, he had attacked my belief system and, I felt, me personally.

We were together sixteen hours a day during the trip. My description of our road trip reflects the anger I felt with finally having to accept my Parkinson's and peripheral neuropathy. Had I been home with Joy, I probably would have directed most of my anger at her.

If Jim comes off in these pages looking like a jerk, it is because everything I wrote at that time was tinged with anger. To sugarcoat my feelings toward Jim at that period of my illnesses' progression would be a disservice to my readers, many of whom I suspect have experienced a similar process of grieving over the loss of a close friend or family member or the advancement of a progressive disease.

After I thought I had climbed out of my funk I told him how I felt. He said he felt awful about it. He wrote several long emails of apology. Each time, I replied something to the effect of "Not to worry. I'm over it." But each time I responded in this manner I lied to Jim, and to myself. In truth, I wasn't over it yet.

After several months, though, I began to see the trip from a completely different perspective. I had begun to realize for the first time that my diseases affected me in significant ways on a daily basis. I needed to be careful about what I ate, how hard I pushed myself when exercising, and how much effort I gave to the charitable organizations I worked with. I held to my belief system but now understood that, as helpful as it might be, it would not enable me to skate through life, pretending there was nothing wrong with me.

Since learning of my Parkinson's six years earlier, I had brushed it aside as something that might affect me later in life but for now was nothing to worry about. When I had called my sister Edythe to tell her about my diagnosis she started to cry. Her reaction startled me. Why didn't she understand that my diseases were "no big deal?" I tried to console her, but to no effect. She said she had to hang up. She was too upset to talk about it.

By then I had already become an expert at denying my diseases affected me in more than a superficial manner—nothing I couldn't handle by thinking about them in the right way. But after this trip I could no longer deny my diseases were a "big deal." It had taken me several months of processing and a deep funk to bring my understanding of this truth from a purely intellectual to an emotional level.

It had been so much easier to simply blame Jim. But I knew now that Jim did not owe me an apology; I owed him an expression of deep gratitude. He had given me a most valuable gift—the gift of friendship. Who would have blamed him if he'd dropped me off at the Rapid City airport after I had caused us to stay an extra night in Jackson Hole and almost gotten us killed in Yellowstone? His rant on abortion, same-sex marriage, capital punishment, and so forth seemed harsh at the time, but in retrospect was milder than many of the debates I had in college about these topics. But far more important, Jim demonstrated real friendship. More than just giving the feedback on my belief system I'd requested, he talked with me for hours at a time about questions regarding God, morality, and belief. But most important, he was always there for me. It must have been hard for him to discover how far his old running buddy's illnesses had progressed. And yet with a matter-of-factness that masked his grace, he helped me when I needed help but left me alone when I didn't.

In the aftermath of this trip I not only started to come to grips with my illnesses—yes, they are a big deal—but also learned an important truth. I will need the love of my friends and family to handle my illnesses in a way I can be proud of.

· · · · · · · · ·

Lest one think our friendship is a one-way relationship, Jim told me several months after the trip that I had helped him, too. He needed to play out the strident elements of his new Catholic faith, to make sense of his new-found belief system. I could easily have bailed out of the arguments. But I was willing to fight back, even in my weakened state. Jim needed more than a sounding board; he needed someone to actively challenge him. And I unwittingly played that role for him. In that way, he said, I had demonstrated the Divine he had been trying to say is within all of us.

The trip was indeed one of discovery, but not in the way I had expected or hoped for. Circumstances dictated I finally come to terms with my illnesses. The wall of denial I had built around myself stone-by-stone and brick-by-brick began first to crack and then to crumble. And with it, so did my self-confidence.

That my friendship with Jim survived this trip and has since grown stronger is testament to the love we feel for our families and long-time friends but rarely acknowledge. When I am feeling lonely I often think this about this trip and the conversations Jim and I had afterwards. It helps to remind me that I am not alone in this world. People really do care.

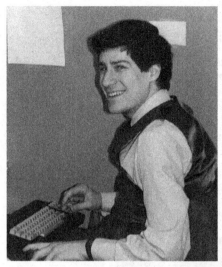

Taking a break from work. In my first job. I was a geek and proud of it (note the vest).

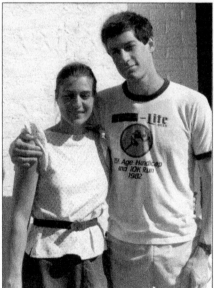

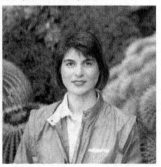

Joy, Honolulu, 1989

Ready to take on the world

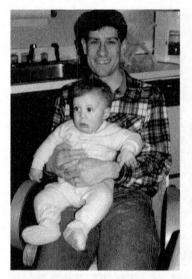 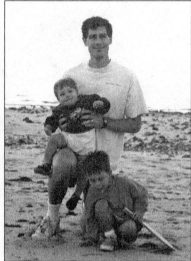

Proud papa of 1   Proud Papa of 2

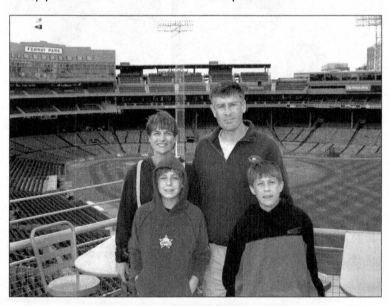

Family dream trip to Fenway Park during the golden years

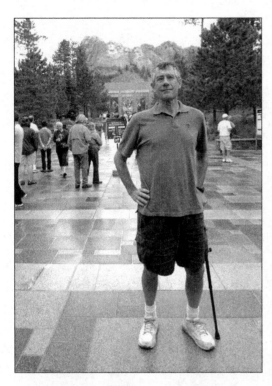

Still taking on the world,
but now with a cane

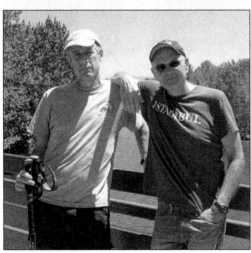

With my friend Jim on our
cross-country trip

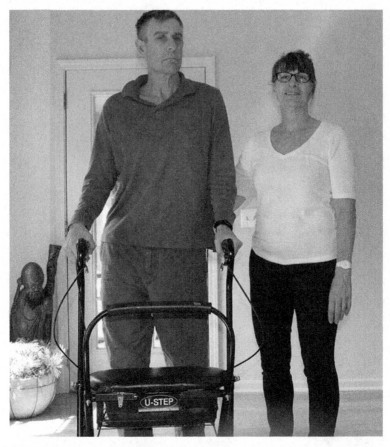

The Wife of the Century and my chariot

CHAPTER 22
ACCEPTANCE

It's Just Emotions

"Where is the rage, the fear, the grief?" people ask me incredulously when I tell them how I cope with my three diseases. "These emotions cannot stay repressed forever; at some point they have to bubble to the surface," a friend I had shared my belief system with challenged me.

I have wondered about this question myself. Why don't I feel the losses I have experienced the way others do? Am I incapable of feeling normal human emotions or have I just repressed them, leaving them somewhere deep in my subconscious? After a considerable amount of introspection and some research on the effects of Parkinson's, I think I have at least a partial answer. The answer is complicated; several forces have combined to dampen my emotions.

I learned from my research that Parkinson's itself provides a small part of the answer. To quote from a scholarly article I found on the Internet site http://brain.oxford-journal.org, "Our findings of attenuated startle reactivity to aversive stimuli add to the growing literature on emotional changes associated with Parkinson's Disease." In other words, Parkinson's itself causes a dampening of emotions, especially negative emotions that result from adverse events—like having three chronic, progressive medical conditions at age fifty-three.

Also providing a small part of the answer is the simple fact that I am now well into my fifties and, like most people, do not experience highs or lows as powerfully as I did in my youth. The way I react when I watch a Red Sox game is a case in point. I used to hang on every pitch, howling in agony or delight depending on the outcome. I recall game six of the 1986 World Series against the Mets—I was twenty-eight years old at the time. As the Mets began their comeback, I screamed at the TV, jumped up and down and threw pillows around the room. It took every ounce of control I had not to smash my TV screen after the ball went through Bill Buckner's legs, sealing the Red Sox fate. The following day, my next door neighbor told me how I had amused him as he watched my temper tantrum through the window. The Red Sox's collapse in that World Series depressed me for weeks afterwards.

Now I enjoy a Red Sox game more when they win than when they lose, but my disappointment after a loss is fleeting. As far back as 2003, a few months shy of my forty-sixth birthday, the Red Sox suffered another devastating loss—this time to the hated Yankees—when Brett Boone hit a walk-off home run in the 11th inning of game seven of the American League Championship Series. The loss upset me, but I did not run around the room during the game throwing pillows like a maniac and it took me only a few days to get over the loss.

The larger part of the answer to my question, though, is that for as long as I can remember I have suffered from a fourth disease: depression. I have never experienced the debilitating hopelessness and futility that William Styron describes in his memoir, *Darkness Visible*, that eventually led him to take his own life. Mine has been more like a low-grade fever that occasionally spikes, but has never become life-threatening.

I have been around the block a few times when it comes to dealing with depression. Along the way, I have learned strategies to cope with it. As an adolescent I learned I could defuse some of my anger by running as hard as I could, until the physical pain overtook my mental anguish. I also discovered that a long, slow run often helped me to sort out whatever problems were troubling me. I didn't realize it at the time, but running was a form of meditation. Only recently, I learned how to practice mindful meditation, now another strategy in my bag of tricks.

In my late twenties I went to a therapist for the first time. I expected to lay on a couch and tell him how my mother had treated me badly and my father had abandoned me. But he was not interested in any of that. Instead he taught me how to use Cognitive Behavioral Therapy.

I now instinctively use these strategies to mute the negative emotions I feel as a result of my three other diseases. Having lived with depression for too long to worry about the stigma associated with the disease, I also get by with a little help from my friends. And since learning I have Parkinson's, I have received talk therapy at least twice a month.

Ironically, my lifelong battle with depression has given me tools to control the negative thoughts that, unchecked, could lead to the rage, fear, and grief that some people expect me to feel. In a sort of virtuous circle, a lifetime of living with depression has helped me to become less depressed by my medical condition than I otherwise would be.

. . . .

All that said, I must admit that I also repress my emotions. I can now see that my habit of automatically going into planning mode is a defense mechanism I learned as a child to distract my mind from the hurt and anger I often felt. When my mother threatened to kick me out of the house, my mind turned to the logistics of living out of my car, the planning temporarily crowding out the despair and anger I might otherwise have felt.

Figuring it All Out

I thought I had it all figured out. I had developed a belief system that helped me to understand how it was possible to be stricken with three serious diseases in my early fifties despite living a healthy lifestyle. Instead of dwelling on "Why me?" I got on with my life. I also had developed a Zen-like ability to live in the present. I avoided thinking about the future and I serenely accepted my losses.

Since the age of fourteen, I had defined myself as a runner and now I could no longer run. *No big deal,* I convinced myself, *I can ride my bike and do power walks instead.* I had also defined myself by my work, but had gone into forced retirement at age fifty-three. Again, not a problem; I accomplished more working a few hours a week as a board member for not-for-profit organizations than I did working fifty-plus hours a week at my last job.

My belief system also gave me a moral code to live by. I knew what I must do and I did it well. Always busy, I found that helping others helped me as well. Finally, after a lifetime of struggling with the demons of my childhood, I was at peace with myself. And best of all, I had written it all down so other people could benefit from my experiences.

Since I went on full disability in March 2011, people from all walks of life—my neighbors, former colleagues at work, fellow board members at the not-for-profits, the new friends I made at Panera's—have expressed admiration for the positive, upbeat demeanor they say I exude. A few people that hardly know me have gone so far as to tell me they think I am a hero and a truly special person. Jim has praised me for carrying myself with grace and dignity. At times, I feel as if I have been anointed the poster child for how someone with a progressive disease can live a productive and meaningful life.

I'm not really a poster child. At least once a week Joy wakes up bleary-eyed to tell me how I awakened her as I screamed and cursed in my dreams. During the day, as I busy myself with activities, I remain positive and upbeat. But in the evening, especially after a bad day of neuropathy pain, I sometimes find myself having the same negative thoughts I believed I had learned to avoid. *How much worse will the pain get?* I worry. *Will I need to use narcotics and become addicted to them?* My word retrieval problem has become noticeably worse and I have become increasingly forgetful. *Are these early signs of dementia?* I fret, even though my doctors told me they are not.

Am I a fraud? Yes, my belief system, moral code and coping strategies have helped me enormously. They motivate me to do the things that keep me busy and feeling positive during the day. But how can I offer them up as an example for others to follow when they sometimes help so little at night? Each word of praise makes me feel more like a fraud. I also started thinking, *So what. My belief system has helped me so far, but what I thought was a gale-force wind was really a light breeze. How will I react when my medical condition starts to make a real difference?* My doubts would continue to grow before I would begin to find an answer.

A Man's Gotta Know His Limitations

My therapist has reminded me that my medical condition has already made a huge difference in my life and I am coping with it quite well. And Joy reassures me that everyone, even people without three chronic, progressive diseases, can have an occasional bad day. She tells me I have set a high standard for myself and I should not expect to live up to it every minute of every day. She suggests maybe the real key to coping with my illnesses is to accept that I will have both good and bad days, I cannot anticipate when the bad days will come, but I can be sure that they will come.

This I Believe—Redux

Good and bad luck. What role do they play in our lives? People often say—as a rebuke to those who complain about their luck and as a palliative to those who have experienced a tragedy—good and bad luck even out in the end. Taken literally, they mean that over a lifetime, people have equal amounts of good and bad luck. Or to be more precise and put it in mathematical terms, they implicitly mean that if a positive (for good luck) or negative (for bad luck) value could be put on the importance of luck on each event in one's life, the total impact of good luck and bad luck on their lives would exactly equal each other, effectively cancelling each other out.

I believe the randomness of events that affect our lives—like a chance encounter that leads to a long, happy marriage or getting early-onset Parkinson's—is more complicated than that. As individuals, we do not each experience equal amounts of good and bad luck. A joke about the two statisticians who went deer hunting helps to make the point. One statistician missed the deer by ten feet on the right. The other missed by ten feet on the left. The two statisticians rejoiced—on average they had shot the deer.

Imagine that each person's experience with randomness is like one hundred flips of a coin, where heads is good luck and tails is bad luck. The average number of heads for the billions of people who have lived or ever will live is fifty. And a large number of people will get exactly fifty heads—for them, everything does even out in the end. But a much smaller number of extremely lucky people will get a hundred heads. And a similarly small number of extremely unlucky people will get a hundred tails.

My point is that luck does play a role in our lives. The luck we experience represents just one instance of the randomness of the universe. Since we cannot change this, we might as well accept it. In my view of the world, there is no conspiracy or higher being that protects, punishes, or tests us. To paraphrase a common refrain, stuff just happens.

I am not a fatalist, though. I believe strongly that by our actions we put ourselves in a position to have more good or bad luck. Someone who walks down the middle of a busy highway is far more likely to get run over by a truck than someone who uses a sidewalk and looks both ways before crossing the street. And as I frequently remind Alan and Sam, someone who studies hard in school and gets good grades has better odds of getting a well-paying job doing something he likes than someone who chooses not to study hard and gets average grades.

· · · · · · · · ·

How long will I live? I often think about my mortality: how long will I live and what will I leave behind? I expect to die young. My father died at fifty-one and his father died at forty-one. If two data points make a trend and the trend continues, I will live to be sixty-one—that gives me two more years.

Before writing this section, I re-read a letter I had received in December 2011 from one of my disability insurance companies. They offered to give me a lump-sum payment in lieu of the monthly payments they were obligated to give me until December 2022, when I reach my sixty-fifth birthday. I thought this letter might give me some clues about my life expectancy. I knew the sooner they expected me to die, the less they would be willing to offer me in a lump-sum payment. *Perhaps using the information they provided*, I thought, *I can derive an actuarial estimate of how long I am likely to live.*

Calculating the present value of a stream of future payments—like my monthly disability checks—is easily done using Excel or a financial calculator. But the insurance company made the calculation far more complicated by also embedding estimates of my mortality in their formula. The letter states: "We consider mortality factors based on your known medical conditions to determine a mortality rating." The letter goes on to explain that, due to my Parkinson's diagnosis, my mortality rating is twice that of the average individual. As a result, the letter states, "We are willing to offer a lump-sum amount approximately equal to 67 percent of the amount we would offer to the average person."

Obsessed with determining how long the company's actuaries expect me to live, I spent an entire day trying to replicate their calculation. Although not entirely successful, I think I came close. Their calculation considers the probability that, having reached age fifty-four, I will live to be fifty-five. Then if I make it to age fifty-five, it calculates the probability I will live to be fifty-six. And so on. I created a model in Excel structured the same way. Ultimately I was unable to determine an exact age when the company's actuaries expect me to die. But starting with their finding that my policy is worth 67 percent of the same policy held by an average person and using different assumptions regarding the probability of dying at each age, I arrived at sixty as the age when I am most likely to die—only one year off the age I had projected using my father's and grandfather's ages.

I don't fear dying. What I fear most is staying alive past the point where my pain becomes too much or I am unable to think clearly enough to live a productive life. I worry I will reach this point before I have had a chance to leave my mark on the world.

Sometimes I let my fears get the better of me. I allow myself to dwell on them. There have even been times— when my neuropathy pain is at its worst—I find myself wishing I could fall asleep and not wake up again. Then I realize that all these thoughts about dying amount to nothing more than self-pity.

I felt enormous guilt about these feelings until I found solace in Joan Didion's memoir about the sudden death of her husband, *The Year of Magical Thinking*. She writes:

"People in grief think a great deal about self-pity. We worry about it, dread it, scourge our thinking for signs of it …The very language we use when we think about self-pity betrays the deep abhorrence in which we hold it: self-pity is *feeling sorry for yourself*, self-pity is *thumb-sucking*, self-pity is *boo hoo poor me …*"

These words have helped me feel less guilty about my occasional lapses into self-pity. I realize now I don't have to always be the positive upbeat person I show to the public. People may say they admire me for my apparent lack of self-pity. But feeling sorry for myself at times doesn't make me a fraud; it makes me human.

Allowing myself to occasionally wallow in self-pity, however, does not mean giving up. I still do what I must and try my best to do it well. When I first started writing this chapter, it meant "Now." Several years later I am able to do much less. I have resigned from the MAP, PPA, and SCS boards. I work out vigorously several times a week— sometimes more—and I continue to work on my memoir. This project will not end when I complete the manuscript. Next I will need to get my book out to as many people as I can who will benefit from it.

And most important, it means remaining a positive force in Sam's and Alan's lives and helping Joy out as much as I can so she does not have to bear the entire burden of my illness. I must do these things because they give meaning to my life.

I allow myself moments of self-pity, but when I feel like giving up I remind myself how much I still have to offer. I think about Alan and Sam—especially Sam. I know he still needs my guidance, even if he disagrees with everything I tell him. I think about all the people who tell me I handle my illnesses well and I am a special person. I realize I must be contributing something to their lives for them to feel this way about me. And I think about Joy and the loneliness and grief she would feel if she were to lose her life partner.

I make my own luck now no less than I did when I worked hard in college and earned the grades I needed to get accepted to Northwestern, where I met Joy. If all I do is stay at home and feel sorry for myself, the probability is nearly 100 percent that my condition will deteriorate. But if I make the effort to do what I must and do it well—even on the days when I feel lousy—the probability is much greater that I will continue to a live a full and productive life for at least a little bit longer. Maybe long enough to leave a legacy that I can be proud of.

Following are responses to questions in the 2/1/15 Claimant Question-naire and the 2/4/15 Physician's Statement from my neurologist. Joy typed the questionnaire responses shown here because I was not longer able to type easily. The physician's statement provided by my neurologist, which follows, shows the status of my medical condition as of 2/4/15.

Claimant Questionnnaire February 2015 responses

Question 1.

Please describe your most current medical condition or conditions (including the specific limitations that they place on your ability to work.

I suffer from three medical conditions: Lymphoma, Parkinson's disease (PD), and Peripheral Neuropathy (PN). I do not feel any symptoms from the Lymphoma. Dr. W, my oncologist, tells me that the cancer is "indolent," which means that it is growing very slowly. He has put me on a "wait and watch" program. I get a CT scan every nine months; as long as Dr. W does not see significant growth of the cancer from one CT scan to the next he will not give me any treatment.

MY PD and PN are both progressive diseases and both have advanced significantly over the last 18 months. The symptoms of these diseases usually, but do not always, act in concert with each other. By that I mean that my PN is usually at its worst during my PD off periods. I have all the same PD symptoms that I had 18 months ago, but they have all become more intense. And I have some new symptoms.

My dyskinesia and/or tremors now make eating from a plate a major challenge. I can still eat by myself, but it now takes considerably longer than it had before. Food falling off of my fork as I raise it to my mouth can be both frustrating and embarrassing.

I have had to significantly curtail my driving due to dyskinesia (during my "on" periods) and neuropathy pain (during my "off" periods). My dyskinesia causes me to swerve back and forth—so far I have been able to contain the swerving to my own lane, so I continue to drive short distances when I cannot find someone to drive for me. I try to avoid driving during neuropathy pain episodes unless it is absolutely necessary. The three or four times I have had to do this over the last six months I have used back roads and have stopped to rest every five minutes or so. My night vision has deteriorated to the point where I no longer drive at all at night. I expect that I will no longer have a driver's license well before I complete this form 18 months from now.

My handwriting is now illegible most of the time. I often have to write words two or three times before they are recognizable. My typing is extremely slow, with lots of errors.

I am finding it considerably harder to concentrate on a task than I had to 18 months ago and I am unable to multi-task. Extreme fatigue also remains a problem for me, especially in the afternoon. I lie in bed for at least two hours most afternoons.

My balance has continued to deteriorate, but I am more careful now—for example, I use a walker in the bathroom at night—which has limited my falls to about three or four times a month. I have been lucky not to get seriously injured during any of these falls.

I also have experienced diminished cognitive abilities over the last 18 months. Of greatest concern is a word-finding problem, which causes me to stop in the middle of sentences while I try to find the right word.

The condition that has had the greatest impact on me over the last 18 months has been the increased frequency and intensity of my peripheral neuropathy episodes. I feel an underlying level of neuropathy pain of about three to four on the 10-point self-reporting pain scale throughout the day. I can stand and walk (with a cane) when the pain is at this level, but I need to stay off my feet as much as possible to limit the pain I know I will feel starting at 8:00 to 9:00 p.m. every evening. The evening pain episodes frequently hit seven to 7.5 on the 10-point scale. At this level of pain I need my wife to help me get ready for bed.

I also experience pain episodes of this magnitude or greater two or three times a week during the day, These episodes are more likely to happen on days after I have not slept well, but otherwise I cannot predict when they will come, how painful they will be or how long they will last.

A neuropathy episode of 7.5 to eight on the ten-point pain scale nearly incapacitates me. I need to lie on my back in bed with a large pillow to raise my feet. All I can do that is semi-productive is read and make short phone calls. These episodes usually last for one to two hours, but can last for as long as six hours as or little as 45 minutes.

Question 2.

Please list all of the types of activities you do during the course of a typical day. What do you specifically do from the time you arise in the morning until you retire at night? Do you require assistance with any of your daily activities?

After a roughly two-hour evening routine that includes flossing and brushing my teeth, going to the bathroom, showering, setting out my pills and clothes for the next day, I am ready to go to sleep by 10:00 p.m. Within the last two months I have needed my wife to set out my pills and clothes because my neuropathy pain has been too intense for me to perform these activities by myself.

On a good morning I wake up at about 7:00 a.m., having gotten nine hours of sleep. I try not to think about the neuropathy pain I will feel for the next one to 1½ hours as my meds take effect. I slowly get out of bed to start the new day. At least as often I wake up at about the same time after a restless night of tossing, turning and worrying. On these days getting out of bed is a struggle physically and emotionally.

I continue to do most of the same activities I have always done: walk, read, send e-mails, talk on the phone, etc. But my ability to do these activities had diminished significantly over the last eighteen months. For example, I can still walk short distances but I can no longer power walk. I started using a cane not long after completing this form the last time and now I rarely leave my house without it. In addition, I used to help with household tasks such as laundry, dishes and talking out the garbage but I can no longer perform them due to intense foot pain and poor balance.

If I am feeling well I drive five minutes to Panera's, where I spend a couple of hours talking to friends, reading and writing. My writing has slowed considerably, partly because my handwriting has become illegible and my typing has slowed, but also because I am finding it hard to concentrate on a task for very long.

When I can I spend the rest of the morning running errands, visiting one of my many health care providers and/ or paying bills. Then, after eating the lunch my wife prepares for me, I spend the next several hours in bed reading and napping.

Before dinner, if I am not suffering from a PN pain episode, I exercise. During the warm weather I prefer to ride my bike (since last summer I have not gone out of my neighborhood because my swerving makes it too dangerous to ride on busy streets. In the colder months I ride a stationary bike. (More below on bike riding.)

Depending on my wife's schedule we eat a meal she has prepared at home or go to a nearby restaurant. She always drives both ways. If she needs to pick something up at a store on the way home, I wait in the car so that I can rest my feet. By the time we have finished eating and are home it is close to 8:00 p.m. and time to start preparing for the next day.

Question 3.
Please provide the following information about the condition causing your disability. Next to any Activity of Daily Living (ADL) please place the number shown next to the statement that most accurately reflects your ability/inability to perform each of them.

I cannot perform any of the listed tasks independently when I an "off" or having a bad neuropathy pain episode. Otherwise, I can do the following:

I can don my apparel but I need help with fasteners. I need to sit on a step rather than the edge of the bed or on a chair when dressing, so I do not fall.

I can feed myself but I frequently spill on my clothes and myself. I use covered cups to avoid spilling when drinking.

I have mild to moderate incontinence which requires me to wear underwear liners.

Most nights I need my wife to supervise me in the shower for safety. I have a seat in the shower as well to provide additional safety.

I have experienced mild cognitive impairment over the last 18 months. When I am tired or am experiencing a bad neuropathy pain episode, I often get confused doing what used to be the simplest of tasks, like adding a tip to a restaurant bill.

Question 4.
What kinds of hobbies or social/community activities did you engage in prior to your disability?

Activities I did before my disability included volunteer work for charitable organizations, running, hiking, playing catch, bicycling, and going to movies and concerts.

I have had to stop doing volunteer work for charitable organizations because I find it too taxing to drive to the office where the meeting is held, stay attentive for the entire meeting and then drive home. I have tried calling in for meetings, but that has proven to be ineffective. Also, I haven't had the energy to keep up with all the back and forth e-mails.

I no longer play catch, walk for exercise, or run. I still go to movies but the last few times I have felt intense neuropathy pain by the end of the movie. I no longer go to concerts as the normal start time of about 8:00 p.m. is too late for me.

Three months ago my neurologist referred me to the Pedaling for Parkinson's research program. I joined the clinical study, where I ride a stationary bike with supervision and assistance three day a week for forty minutes at a time. The intent of the study is to identify the positive impact that bike riding, under certain conditions, can have on the progression of PD.

Since becoming disabled I have taken up writing. My wife got me an iPad which has a speech-to-text feature. This has made the writing process more efficient but does not fully compensate for my challenges with word finding and language formulation.

A caveat to the list of activities above is that I cannot do any of these activities during my "down" time.

FUNCTIONAL CAPABILITIES

Please complete the applicable portion of this section based on your most recent clinical assessment.
In a general workplace environment the patient is able to:

	Sit	Stand	Walk
Number of hours at a time	2 hr	15 min	30 min
Total hours / day			

Please circle / check the frequency that the patient can perform the following activities:

R = Right L = Left B = Bilateral		Never	Occasionally (1-33%)	Frequently (34-67%)	No Restriction
Lift / carry 1 to 10 lbs.		R L B	R L B	R L B	R L (B)
Lift / carry 11 to 20 lbs.		R L B	R L B	R L (B)	R L B
Lift / carry 21 to 50 lbs.		R L B	R L (B)	R L B	R L B
Lift / carry 51 to 100 lbs.		R L (B)	R L B	R L B	R L B
Lift / carry over 100 lbs.		R L (B)	R L B	R L B	R L B
Bending at waist					X
Kneeling / Crouching					X
Driving					X
Reaching only (not load-bearing)	Above shoulder	R L B	R L B	R L B	R L (B)
	At waist / desk level	R L B	R L B	R L B	R L (B)
	Below waist / desk level	R L B	R L B	R L B	R L (B)
Fingering / handling		R L B	R L (B)	R L B	R L B

Is the patient's vision impaired? ☐ Yes ☒ No   If "Yes," please describe the extent of the impairment. _____

Best corrected vision: R _____   L _____

Does the patient have a psychiatric / cognitive impairment? ☐ Yes ☐ No   If "Yes," please describe the extent of the impairment and its etiology:

YES, PAIN LIMITS ABILITY TO FOCUS ON WORK UNDER STRESS

Expected duration of any current restriction(s) or limitation(s) listed above LIFETIME

Do you believe the patient is competent to endorse checks and direct the use of the proceeds? ☒ Yes ☐ No

PHYSICIAN INFORMATION

Provider's Name:	Telephone Number:
Degree: MD Specialty: Neurology	Fax Number:
License Number:	Social Security Number or EIN Number:
Street Address:	Ann Arbor State: MI Zip Code: 48101
Signature:	Date signed: 1/26/17

LC-71374 (LTD FR)   Page 2 of 2   04/2012

CHAPTER 23
A VERY PARKIE DAY

S ince shortly after learning of my Parkinson's diagnosis I have used the moniker "Parkie" to refer to
myself and others afflicted with the disease. I first
saw "Parkie" in the book *The First Year—Parkinson's Disease: An Essential Guide for the Newly Diagnosed*, by Jackie
Hunt Christensen. I liked the term "Parkie" because it
conveyed an element of fun and playfulness, of not taking myself or the disease too seriously. Calling myself a
Parkinsonian or simply "Someone with Parkinson's" would
have made the disease sound ominous, something to fear.
But in the beginning, I thought I had nothing to worry
about with Parkinson's. *"Sure, it will cause problems in the
distant future,"* I thought, *"but for now it is no more than a
minor inconvenience."*

I had joked, even bragged, about being a Parkie. My
Parkiness—a rhetorical flourish I added to Christensen's
"Parkie"—made me a hero in the neighborhood just for
doing the things I had always done for relaxation and
enjoyment: running, riding my bike, and going for walks.
My Parkinson's even seemed to make me a more interesting, more popular person. Everyone wanted to get to know
the guy with Parkinson's who had such a positive outlook.

Not long after becoming a Parkie, I learned I also had
peripheral neuropathy, a disease that causes damage to the
part of the nervous system that affects the feet and hands.
People experience peripheral neuropathy in many different

ways. To me it feels like the pain you get when you warm up from frostbite. My neuropathy pain comes in episodes of varying length, intensity, and frequency. I call these episodes Parkie attacks (although the neurologist I saw when they started told me they were independent of my Parkinson's). My Parkie attacks were no more than a curiosity when they started but have become steadily worse over time. Now, six years after my peripheral neuropathy diagnosis, the pain can sometimes be more than I can bear for an hour or more.

When my Parkie attacks and Parkinson's symptoms were mild, I could hold on to the illusion these diseases would not have much impact on my life. I glided through, Zen-like, calmly looking through the rear-view window to see what I had lost, but rarely turning around to see what the diseases had in store for me. In my own little world of denial, Parkinson's and peripheral neuropathy hadn't affected me yet.

The first cracks in the artifice of denial that I had so carefully constructed became visible during my road trip with Jim. Whenever I had looked at myself in the mirror, I saw the same healthy, athletic person I had always known—a little grayer around the temples, but otherwise the same. But I could not deny the look of concern that reflected back at me from Jim's eyes when he had to take me to the emergency room, or when he saw me have some of my especially painful Parkie attacks. My magic mirror of denial had lied. I learned not only that my Parkinson's and peripheral neuropathy had already taken a toll on me, but that if I did not respect my diseases, I could easily end up in the hospital, or worse. Now, several years after my road trip with Jim, I finally recognize my Parkinson's for what it is: to paraphrase Christensen, it is a neurological disorder that causes progressive loss of nerve cell function in the part of the brain that controls muscle movement. Many of its symptoms, at first imperceptible, eventually become debilitating. My symptoms have galloped past the mild stage and are now racing headlong toward life-altering. The moniker, Parkie, however playful, no longer evokes quite as much fun as it used to.

Parkinson's and peripheral neuropathy have affected me in ways big and small. I no longer play a role in the charitable organizations I supported. I rarely stay out past nine, as that is the witching hour when my neuropathy pain often transitions from annoying to so intense that walking from the sink where I brush my teeth to the shower is a major achievement. And now, whenever I schedule a meeting or appointment it is with the caveat that I may have to cancel if my neuropathy pain gets out of control.

The other symptoms are easier for others to see. Now when I sit down for a meal in the late afternoon or early evening I often look like a child out of control. My arms flail this way and that while my torso moves from side-to-side, my head practically touching the table with each back and forth movement. If I concentrate extra-hard I can stop moving, but usually after a few minutes my concentration lapses and I start up again. The movements, called dyskinesia, are a side-effect of Sinemet. The more Sinemet I take, the better able I am to control my Parkinson's symptoms—and my neuropathy pain—but the less able I am to control dyskinesia.

As hard as I try, I now rarely complete a meal without getting some of it on me. I have to carefully plan my moves to avoid making a mess whenever I go to a friend's house. I now routinely check the placement of my drink to ensure it is outside striking distance of my elbows. Red wine at a dinner party is a Parkie no-no.

To Joy and my doctors, most worrisome of the Parkinson's symptoms is my gradual loss of balance. A bad fall, Joy frequently reminds me, can cause serious injury. I fall about two or three times a week and have at least eight to ten near falls each day. Fortunately, I have been nimble enough to fall the right way and not get hurt. At home, if I feel myself losing balance I quickly find a wall to bounce off of, a chair to sit in, or a couch or bed to dive onto.

I was able to get away with bouncing off walls and diving onto furniture for only so long. Now, I am falling more frequently. My poor balance is exacerbated by a symptom that is a hallmark of Parkinson's: smallness and slowness of movement. I can easily spot someone with advanced Parkinson's. He is the (usually elderly) man barely shuffling along, his feet practically touching each other. I look a lot like this guy when I am having one of my bad neuropathy attacks. That is what Jim saw when I inched toward his car after the gondola ride down the mountain near Jackson Hole, Wyoming.

Another noticeable symptom of Parkinson's is the loss of volume and tenor in a Parkie's voice. Mine has become softer and more monotonic as Parkinson's has advanced. I wouldn't have noticed the change myself had Joy, a speech pathologist, not brought it to my attention. She often tells me when we are at a restaurant that she can barely hear me. At her urging, I raise my voice to the point where I think people at every other table must be able to hear me.

But Joy assures me that they cannot. My louder voice is just right for us to have a normal conversation.

Occasionally during a meeting someone will ask me to speak up so everyone can hear me. I have to admit I sometimes get an ego boost when people have to lean in to hear me speak—like the insurance commercial: "When Ira speaks, people listen." But slipping back to reality, I realize that if my voice becomes much softer it will prevent me from participation in some conversations. I cannot imagine too many experiences that would be more frustrating than being unable to communicate because people cannot hear me.

I cannot stop my Parkinson's from progressing, but I can take some measures to slow it down. Not long after I retired, my neurologist referred me to a physical therapist who taught me a series of exercises called BIG therapy. The program focuses on making repeated large movements. It has been proven BIG can forestall the shrinkage in body movements if practiced regularly.

At about the same time, Joy put me through a similar therapy for my voice, called LOUD Therapy. Joy taught me a series of exercises that involved speaking much louder than my normal voice. Similar to BIG therapy, LOUD therapy has been proven to help Parkies maintain their voices if they practice the exercises regularly.

These therapies have been available to me for several years. But I haven't used them much. I didn't think I needed to. For as long as I could, I continued to do the same workouts I had done in recent years: power walking, riding my bike during the warm weather months and my stationary hand bike during the rest of the year, and occasionally even running. But only occasional BIG and LOUD exercises. The progression of Parkinson's that I could have averted by doing BIG and LOUD therapy is incalculable.

The symptom that scares me the most is dementia. According to the Henry Ford Health System website, early-onset Parkies like me have about a 50 percent chance of developing dementia. With Parkinson's, symptoms of dementia usually begin to appear after about ten to fifteen years regardless of the Parkie's age at onset. I started to exhibit signs of Parkinson's about four years before getting my diagnosis. That means I should be in the time frame when dementia signs start to appear.

Dementia comes on very gradually, so it's hard to tell whether what looks like an early sign of dementia really is dementia. We all have our senior moments. I frequently walk into a room to get something and by the time I get there have forgotten what I went into the room for. But Joy does the same thing. Are we both suffering from early dementia?

With all this to worry about, I thought I had kept my equanimity fairly well. That is until I had a very Parkie day....

A Very Parkie Day, 2012

The day started off well enough. I had gotten a good night's sleep and felt rested. I wolfed down a large bowl of oatmeal and a banana for breakfast, hurrying to get to the Non-profit Enterprises at Work (NEW) Center for Michigan Ability Partner's (MAP)'s board retreat well before its scheduled 8 a.m. start. I never knew how much my neuropathy pain and dyskinesia from Parkie meds would cause me to move around so I wanted to get there early enough to find a place to sit with plenty of leg room.

I felt a sense of déjà vu as I drove down the steep driveway to the NEW Center. I had spent countless hours in this building during my first two years on the Partners in Personal Assistance (PPA) board. I strode into the building, climbed the steps to the second floor, and quickly found my way to the South Conference Room. As I entered, I looked through the windows across the room and took in the familiar view of railroad tracks running alongside the building, the strip of greenbelt, and the Huron River off in the distance. Then I turned back to the inside wall of the room and found one of the few places where the legs from the folding tables wouldn't get in the way of my own legs. I spread out a notebook and Board Retreat materials to mark my territory, grabbed one of the hard plastic chairs, and sat down.

For several minutes I sat in the room by myself. That gave me time—too much time—to reminisce about the past. I recalled how at the PPA meetings I was the guy who everyone looked to for answers, how I was the unofficial chair of every board committee, and how I had been asked several times to take over as Board Chairman.

My thoughts then turned to MAP. When I joined MAP's board the first time, three years earlier, the organization was in a state of turmoil. The founder and twenty-five-year CEO had abruptly resigned a month before I started. Jan, the Director of Operations and long-time number-two person on MAP's staff, seemed to me to be the obvious person for the CEO job, but several board members opposed her. After a formal recruitment process that dragged on for several months, Jan finally won the job. I played a major role in swaying the final vote her way despite having only recently joined the board.

Not more than a month later, MAP's board president resigned. By then I had earned recognition as one of the key people to include whenever we had a difficult and/or important issue to discuss. Jan, the departing Board President, and the Board Treasurer asked if I would take over as Board President, but not wanting the attention the position would bring, I declined. I agreed instead to take on the unofficial role of co-Board President. My responsibilities were to provide direction to Jan and act as the liaison between her and the rest of the board. I did not have a title, but I had become Jan's de-facto job coach/mentor.

Those were the glory days. In addition to the work I did for MAP and PPA, I co-wrote a strategic plan for a third non-profit agency and led a fourth through a partnering strategy process. Whatever organization I joined, I quickly became a leader.

• • • • • • • • •

I glanced at the clock on the wall and saw it was already 7:49. That snapped me back to the present. I had been day-dreaming for a good ten minutes. Seconds later Jan appeared at the door. We exchanged greetings and started a conversation but were interrupted by another board member who arrived right behind her. For the next few minutes the rest of the group, which included some senior staff as well as the board members, straggled in. I stood up to greet the few people whose faces I recognized but otherwise stayed put and observed as the other meeting attendees casually put their stuff down at an open spot and mingled with the rest of the crowd.

My mind drifted off again as I waited for the meeting to begin. I stewed about having almost no involvement in the planning for this retreat. No one had sought out my advice. My role was limited to answering a survey that Greg, the current Board President, had sent out to all board members. I no longer had special status on the board—and it bugged me.

I realized, though, that I no longer had a legitimate claim to special status. In at least this one respect, non-profit charitable organizations are similar to for-profit companies: status is earned by accomplishment and what matters most is what you have done lately.

I sensed the other board members viewed me as an old lion, once a key player but no longer with much to contribute. At least that was how I felt about myself. Since re-joining the board I hadn't participated in any fund-raising activities. My only contribution had been to serve on the Finance Committee. But strategy was my strong suit and that would be the focus of the retreat. This would be my day to shine. I just hoped my Parkiness didn't get in the way.

Greg woke me from my reverie when he announced last call for coffee before we got started. I ambled over to the coffee machine and poured myself a cup. I made sure not to fill it too high so as not to spill any on the way back to my seat. I spilled some anyway, putting a stain on my freshly-cleaned khaki pants.

Greg called the meeting to order. He turned our attention to the agenda, which he had emailed to us a few days earlier. He explained that Jan and he had three main goals for the retreat: to identify MAP's top strategic priorities, to educate board members on their responsibilities, and to give them an opportunity to see some of our housing sites. He passed the gavel on to Karen, NEW's Vice President for Board Development. Karen facilitated the meeting for the rest of the morning.

She started by dividing us into four groups of four or five people each. Then she asked each group to develop a consensus on MAP's top five priorities and to nominate a spokesperson to share its conclusions with the rest of the meeting attendees. She gave us twenty minutes to complete the assignment. I would have liked to have demonstrated some leadership by taking on the role of scribe and spokesperson for our group. But concerned about my inability to write legibly and my quickly worsening word-finding problem, I hung back and let somebody else speak for our group.

After all the groups had reported their findings, Karen summarized the results. Then she gave us another assignment. This time we were to identify the qualities we should look for in a board member. Once again I let somebody else be the spokesperson for our group.

Following these group exercises, we took a short break for lunch—pizza, salad, and drinks. As I approached the food line I made a strategic decision. I would start with salad and then come back for pizza. Having less on my plate at any one time would reduce the chances of spilling and drawing unwanted attention. Careful to look straight ahead during the entire trip, I managed to bring my plate to the table without incident. I didn't look for anyone to talk to, as eating alone enabled me to devote my full attention to not making a mess.

My efforts went for naught. I had strewn pieces of lettuce and tomato all over the place. I cleaned up my droppings as discreetly as possible and headed back to the buffet to get some pizza and a drink.

I put a piece of pizza on a paper plate and carefully filled a cup with water. Then, with the plate in one hand and the cup in the other, I started to make my way back to my seat. But before I got there, I ran into Greg. He stopped me and asked what I thought of the retreat so far. Stuck in the "Spill Zone," I told him I thought it was going great. But Greg wanted more than a one-word answer, so I started to elaborate, ever careful not to spill the water in my cup. Greg seemed to be paying attention until suddenly his gaze shifted and he pointed to my right hand. Confused, I looked to see what he was pointing at. But by then it was too late. My slice of pepperoni pizza had slid off the plate and landed on the floor, sauce side down. Greg wandered off to another conversation while I picked up my mess and hurried to the garbage pail to rid myself of it. Then I went back to the buffet, grabbed another piece of pizza and safely brought it back to my spot. My face stinging with embarrassment, I ate the pizza with my head down to ward off anyone else who might consider striking up a conversation with me.

After lunch, Karen delivered a presentation about the duties and responsibilities of board members of not-for-profit organizations. I had heard this presentation before. Board members have many responsibilities, Karen intoned, but most important is to raise funds for the organization.

Greg took over at this point and reminded us he had asked each of us to create a fundraising plan with goals for the year—what fundraising events would we sponsor and/or host? To whom would we make direct appeals and for how much? And so on.

I like asking people for money just slightly more than I enjoy having my teeth drilled. In the past, contributions of my time had been more than enough. I felt my whole body become tense when Greg announced that all but one board member—me—had submitted his fundraising plan for the upcoming fiscal year.

Greg concluded the meeting with a short rah-rah speech. As we got up to leave, Jan reminded us she had scheduled visits to MAP's temporary housing units. These visits were an important part of the retreat. We would get to see first-hand how our efforts helped our clients, mostly veterans of the Iraq and Afghanistan wars with mental health disabilities. MAP provides housing, access to mental health care, training on how to find and keep a job, and several other services that helps vets get back on their feet. Without MAP's involvement, many of them would be living on the street.

Jan offered a ride in MAP's van to anyone who wanted it. Most of the group accepted her offer, but I decided to drive by myself. That would allow me to leave the tour after seeing only two or three sites if I wanted. *I should be able to find the sites easily enough using OnStar*, I reasoned.

With that decision, the truly embarrassing part of my very Parkie day began.

The first house was located on a busy street in a sketchy neighborhood. I couldn't see the numbers on the houses as I sped along just fast enough to keep up with traffic. When OnStar told me I had passed the house I shut it down. I turned around and found a place to park that I thought was close to the MAP house. But I had miscalculated. After a long walk that included at least three stops at wrong addresses, I found the MAP house. Unlike the others on the street, this one had a fresh coat of paint and an immaculate front yard. I knocked and a thin man with a stiff, formal countenance who appeared to be in his late twenties opened the door. I told him I was with the MAP Board of Directors tour and asked him if I was at the right place. He answered, "Yes, it is, sir. The tour started ten minutes ago." Then with a firm, almost too strong hand shake, he introduced himself to me as Robert. I told him my name was Ira Fried.

Robert opened the front door to a common room where two other men, who also appeared to be in their late twenties, sat on a couch watching a Tigers game. Robert introduced me to them as Mr. Fried. Jason and Sam both introduced themselves in what struck me as an overly polite and deferential manner.

Introductions finished, Robert told me the Board of Directors tour had just moved outside to the backyard; I could join it there. I asked if instead I could sit and chat with Jason, Sam, and him until the tour group returned to the house—I thought that by spending some time alone with these MAP clients, I might get to know them a little as individuals. Robert answered, "Yes sir, you may," in a tone that evoked a private answering a general's command. I joined Jason and Sam on the couch while Robert made himself comfortable on a lounge chair. My body jerked back and forth, causing me to almost bump into Jason and Sam several times, but none of the guys gave any indication that they noticed my movements. I tried to make conversation but didn't get much further than small talk about the Tigers and the weather. In retrospect, I think all I accomplished by talking with these three men was to put them on edge.

Soon enough, the other board members returned to the house, assembling in the common room. As they approached, Jason and Sam departed, presumably for the privacy of their bedrooms. Not wanting to be the only person sitting, I got up from the couch and joined my colleagues. Thankfully, Robert stayed and stood next to me. A minute or two later, Jan cleared her throat and continued with the tour. During the three or four minutes that Jan spoke, I lost my balance twice. Both times Robert caught me and prevented me from falling. Unfortunately, he couldn't prevent everyone else from seeing me almost fall.

As we left the room, I inadvertently glanced at the TV and caught another glimpse of the Tigers game. That gave me an idea. Several months earlier, I had bought six tickets to the Red Sox/Tigers game for the upcoming Sunday afternoon. However, a few days earlier I learned, much to my disappointment, that the Tigers had changed the start time from 1:15 to 8:15 p.m. to accommodate TV coverage. That meant getting home from the game after midnight—well past my bedtime. The tickets had become useless to me. But maybe not to MAP, I thought. Our clients would surely jump at the opportunity to go to a Tigers game. We could do a lottery, to see which six lucky clients would get to go.

After the tour ended I sidled over to Jan to tell her about my idea. She thanked me but not as enthusiastically as I had expected. She explained she would have to work out some challenging logistical issues, like arranging for transportation on short notice. But she said she would give it a try.

I got in my car and looked for the address of the next place on the list. Noticing it was less than two miles from my house, I decided to make this visit the last stop on my tour. Then I had another brainstorm. Instead of driving straight to the temporary housing unit I would first drive home and pick up the tickets so I could give them to Jan.

I got home, grabbed the tickets, and headed to the second tour stop. *It should take me no more than five minutes to get there,* I thought. But nothing came easily for me on my very Parkie day. I could not find the damned building. I drove back and forth along a four block stretch where I knew it had to be, all the while trying to reach Jan on her cell phone. Finally, Jan called me and directed me to the site. She said she had turned her phone off. I arrived about ten minutes after the tour had ended.

Jan gave me a puzzled look when I gave her the tickets. "You didn't need to give me a printout of the tickets," she said. "All you needed to do was email the file to me." I wanted to make myself invisible. Jan, perhaps sensing my embarrassment, offered to give me a quick private tour of the group home. But I declined. I wanted to get away from anybody associated with MAP as quickly as I could. I went straight home and for the rest of the day wallowed in my Parkiness. The next day Jan told me she had to cancel the lottery due to lack of interest. Our clients didn't want to get home past midnight on a Sunday night any more than I did.

. . . .

My illnesses have continued to progress since my very Parkie day. In retrospect, my attitude, more than my illnesses, made my very Parkie day so memorably bad. I wanted people to treat me as the leader I had once been. But each mishap reminded me I am no longer that person. My glory days are over. So what if I used to run two marathons a year, win the President's Club award for sales achievement every year at work, and spend innumerable hours every week in the backyard playing with my kids. I am no longer that person, either.

It took my very Parkie day to begin to recognize and accept myself as the person I am now, someone who is limited in ways I was not just a short time ago. As Clint Eastwood once said, "A man has gotta know his limitations." ... But a man also has to test his limits occasionally to ensure he doesn't underestimate his capabilities.

An Very Unparkie Day

Summer Camp Scholarships (SCS) had scheduled its annual golf outing to take place just two weeks after the MAP board retreat. I wanted to participate but doubted I could. Wouldn't all my extraneous body movements make it impossible for me to hit the ball? How would I hold up for the four to five hours it takes to play 18 holes? What if I got a bad peripheral neuropathy pain episode while I was out on the course?

I had told Jim about the golf outing and he agreed to come along. I wavered until the night before the tournament when, with Jim's encouragement, I decided to go. The outing was staged as a best ball tournament, in which the foursome agrees on the best lie after each shot and everyone takes their next swing from there. Jim and I knew we had no chance to compete in any foursome that included the two of us. We hoped to play as a twosome so we could ignore the tournament, relax, and just have fun.

We arrived at the golf course at 7:45 for an 8 a.m. start. But at the last moment we were paired up with two other guys, Jason and his father-in-law, Jack. Jim and I murmured to each other before play got underway that Jason and Jack appeared to be regular golfers. We hoped they would not turn out to be hyper-competitive jerks. Jim and I soon learned that our initial impression of Jason and Jack was correct. They played at least twice a week and were accomplished amateur golfers. Jim, the star of our twosome, had played regularly in his teens and early twenties, but only sporadically since then. As for myself, I played putt-putt and hit from the driving range with Alan and Sam now and then when they were young and had played in two SCS golf outings several years earlier. Otherwise I hadn't touched a golf club in over twenty years. My lack of athleticism combined with my unintended Parkie movements made me a noticeably bad player. I doubted I would contribute anything to our foursome.

We drove our carts to the first hole. For no particular reason Jason went first, then Jack, then Jim, then me. On Jason's and Jack's drives you could hear the crack of the club hitting the ball, followed by a whistling sound as the ball soared like a missile toward the pin. Both of their balls landed on the fairway over 250 yards from where we stood. Jim's ball went about 200 yards but landed well off the fairway in the woods.

Finally, my turn came. I took a couple of practice swings, then stood over the ball and prepared to swing. I reminded myself one last time: *you don't need to hit it hard—just make contact.* I didn't want to hit a little dribbler off the end of my club. I wound up, and using the mindfulness skills I had learned, put my full attention on the ball. I swung. Whoosh! I missed it completely. I bent down to pick up my tee, but before I reached it I heard Jack say, "Take another swing."

I asked if he was sure and Jason piped in, "Go ahead. We're just here to have fun."

So I put the ball back on the tee and swung again, this time without all the mental preparation. Whack—a low line drive. My ball stopped rolling about a hundred yards away, on the edge of the fairway. I thought to myself, *This might turn out to be a good day after all.*

I played surprisingly well the rest of the day. I hit the ball solidly on about half of my swings. I even made six shots we used as our best ball—yes, I counted. I almost forgot I was a Parkie. Not until the last three or four holes, when I started to become tired and tremors in both hands made balancing the ball on the tee difficult, did my illnesses slow me down.

Exhausted, I stood over the ball one last time at the 18th tee. This time I wanted to do more than just connect; I wanted to drive the ball far. I reared back and, using all of my remaining strength, swung my driver as hard as I could. Thwack! I watched in amazement as the ball flew down the middle of the fairway, finally stopping 180 yards from where I had teed off. That capped off a very un-Parkie day.

The Banquet

After my Parkie Day, I continued to serve on MAP's board for another six months. I tried to attend in person a couple of times but couldn't do it. The meetings were scheduled for three hours—5 to 8 p.m., once a month. I lacked the stamina to concentrate for more than about two hours, plus that time of day was prime time for neuropathy attacks. So I ended up participating in board meetings mainly by phone.

To paraphrase T.S. Eliot, I left MAP with a whimper, not a bang. When the board president asked me to take responsibility for leading a board planning process, I happily agreed. Several other board members agreed to work with me on the project. It started well enough—I came up with a methodology that would enable us to come up with meaningful results quickly. But as the deadline approached, it became difficult for the committee to meet. We communicated endlessly by email, which soon became overwhelming. I could not keep up and soon lost control of the project. Without a word, another member of the committee assumed my responsibilities.

I told Jan I was no longer up to the task of contributing to MAP as a board member. And that was that.

My tenure on the board officially ended. I quit on good terms, but a small part of me couldn't get over feeling unappreciated. That is, until MAP's 2015 banquet.

When a square envelope from MAP appeared in our mailbox, I barely took notice, discarding it with all the other mail bound for the recycling bin.

When I got a reminder about the banquet requesting an R.S.V.P, I thought, *Why not go? It might be enjoyable.*

On the evening of the banquet, Joy and I dressed up to go, and so did my mother-in-law, who happened to be visiting. What a wonderful evening it turned out to be. After members who had gone through the program were recognized, I thought the awards were over and it was time for the silent auction. Then Jan asked us to stay in our seats just a little bit longer. I was surprised when she called me and two other individuals up to the podium. I was one of the honorees—recognized for my service as a board member from 2011 to 2014.

Jan presented me with a plaque, now hanging in my family room, that shows an antique map depicting the Old and New Worlds. Inscribed in gold calligraphy at the bottom are these words:

Ira Fried
Michigan Ability Partners
Board Member 2011-2014
Thank you for your invaluable support in helping MAP find its way.
We couldn't have done it without
your wisdom and guidance.
February 23,2015

The banquet caused all my negative feelings to melt away. Being recognized for my contributions made all the difference. Having Joy and my mother-in-law there to share in the warmth was the icing on the cake.

CHAPTER 24
CAREGIVER OF THE DECADE

This has been the most difficult chapter of my memoir to write. I want to talk about how Joy is a wonderful person and how our enduring love has kept me strong as I have battled my illnesses. I want to tell the whole world how every time self-doubt has crept into my mind, Joy has restored my confidence. And I want to shout from the rooftops how through it all Joy has managed to be not only a loving wife but also a terrific caregiver.

But each time I've tried to write these words, I've gotten nowhere. I have been unable to write so much as a sentence. Finally I realized what was wrong. I had been too angry to write. My Parkinson's and peripheral neuropathy have seemed to progress at an accelerating pace. I often waste hours waiting for my neuropathy pain episodes to end. I fear I may be losing some of my cognitive abilities. No longer am I able to sit back and serenely watch my capabilities float by into the past. I often get angry now—sometimes at the smallest provocations, sometimes at the world in general, and yes, sometimes at Joy. We argue more now than we did before my PD and PN started ravaging my body. But so far we're managing to make it work. Our relationship is undergoing a difficult transformation: from one of two equal partners to an unbalanced relationship with Joy playing the role of caregiver and me the patient.

All these things I want to say about Joy are true. I don't

know what I would do without her. And that, I think, is the crux of the problem. I sometimes find myself resenting Joy because I need her so much, just as I hated Jim in the moment he rescued me at the hotel during our drive from Portland to Ann Arbor.

Who's in charge here? Now, Joy is in charge. She decides what we need and don't need for the house. If Alan or Sam wants something, they go to her first because they know she will be the final arbiter. Joy goes to all of my doctor appointments. I rarely go to any of hers. Unlike the progression of my diseases, the changes in our relationship have come so gradually that I sometimes don't realize how much my condition has affected it.

One day Joy saw me take an inordinate amount of time to organize my pills for the coming week. She asked if she could do it and I reluctantly accepted her offer. Now organizing my pills is one of the countless tasks Joy does every day to support me.

Joy's ever-changing role has progressed from Wife of the Century to Caregiver of the Decade. Before my PD diagnosis, I had prided myself on being part of a 50/50 relationship. Jim sometimes joked that I was a man of the fifties because I put in long hours at the office, but did very little at home. I insisted I was a man of the eighties because Joy and I made all the big decisions together. I prided myself on being part of an equal partnership with Joy. But after my PD diagnosis I saw that our partnership had been far from equal. Without realizing it, I had been the dominant partner in ways small and large. I paid the check at restaurants, I drove whenever we went somewhere together in a car. I negotiated with the sales manager to agree on a price whenever we made a major purchase.

During our twenties and thirties we moved five times, each time to further my career. We reasoned that, since I made two to three times as much as Joy, I was the primary bread-winner. I did whatever I thought necessary to further my career—extensive travel, sixty-hour work weeks, frequent dinners with colleagues and clients, and so on.

I searched nationally whenever I needed to find a new job. I felt I had to because suitable positions for me were few and far between. Not many companies needed someone with my combination of strategic and quantitative analysis skills, but the few that did fell all over themselves to get me. We moved from Chicago to Minneapolis, Dallas, New York, Stamford, Amherst, and finally to Ann Arbor, all to pursue my career.

How things have changed in the years since my Parkinson's diagnosis.

Jim and I sometimes joke that conversations are all about me. At home it really is all about me most of the time. Sure, I always ask Joy how her day went, and when she comes home from tennis, how she thinks she played. We talk about these things for a while, but the discussion inevitably moves on to my day. I tell her how bad my neuropathy episode(s) had been, how painful they were, how long I had laid in bed incapacitated. I try not to talk about my pain so much, but I can't help myself. My neuropathy pain episodes define my days. They determine how much and what I am able to accomplish. I try not to let them control my mood, but I can't prevent them from having an impact. Joy gets to hear all the negative thoughts I have bottled up all day. All this after a full day of work.

And it does not stop there. I often experience extremely painful episodes in the evening, usually starting at about nine o'clock. At their worst they can make walking just two or three steps excruciatingly painful. So I rely on Joy for everything. "Joy, can you get me some water?" "Joy, can you get me the *Times*? I think I left it on the kitchen table." Joy, can you find my MAP strategy file and put it on the passenger seat of the car? It's in my office, I think in the stack of files on the right-hand corner of my desk." Sometimes even, "Joy, can you pull the blankets over me? It hurts too much for me to do that. Don't forget to fold the blanket and sheet by my ankles."

At least one or two nights a week I wake up moaning from the pain. Joy wakes up, looks at me through her glassy eyes and asks, "What can I do for you?"

Taking care of me is just one of Joy's many responsibilities. I do what I can to help, but still, one by one, she is taking back the chores I have been handling: putting the dishes in the dishwasher and taking them out when they are clean; taking the garbage and recycling down to the end of the driveway every Thursday night and bringing the empty containers back up on Friday afternoon. She had already been doing all of the cooking and 99 percent of the shopping. None of these chores seem like much by themselves but together they can be overwhelming.

Sometimes I get angry at Joy because of the words she says to me in anger. I have not stopped believing that

Joy is an amazing person, a wonderful wife, and a terrific caregiver, but I've come to see she's also not perfect. Just as I have had to accept that my illnesses are real and serious, I've also had to accept that they have put an enormous strain on her. She is doing the best she can.

We have to constantly recalibrate our expectations of each other. How much help do I need and what type? How much of that help is Joy capable of giving? I tend to be optimistic—in denial—about my capabilities. I think I can push myself to the limit. Whenever I ride my bike during the Pedaling for Parkinson's classes, I forget that each time I push myself too hard I wind up lying in bed, enduring neuropathy pain for most of the next two days. I also have a hard time planning for the future. I cannot envision my condition getting any worse.

Joy tends to be pessimistic—a realist—about my condition. She usually does far more for me than I can reasonably expect. She has spoiled me, often getting me something I want—a cup of water, an apple, dental floss, or whatever else I need—before I even think to ask for it. But Joy has also infuriated me at times by underestimating my cognitive and other capabilities. I have never been angrier at Joy than the time she excluded me from an important discussion regarding one of our sons because, she said, I lacked the cognitive ability to contribute to the discussion and my participation would only increase all of our stress.

I tell Joy she looks more beautiful every day, and I mean it. (She jokes that my vision is deteriorating.)

I should have known it at the time, but when I took

the leap of faith to ask Joy to marry me, I leapt over a crack, not a chasm. Joy, on the other hand, may not have realized it at the time, but she leapt over a canyon of faith to say yes.

Following are responses to questions in the 6/27/16 Claimant Questionnaire and the 6/27/16 Physician's Statement from my neurologist.

Joy typed the questionnaire responses shown here. The physician's statement provided by my neurologist shows progression of my medical condition as of 6/27/16.

Claimant Questionnnaire June 2016 responses

Question 1.
Please describe your most current medical condition or conditions (including the specific limitations that they place on your ability to work.

I continue to suffer from Parkinson's and peripheral neuropathy (PN). These are both progressive diseases, which means my symptoms are worsening over time. At this point I am ambulating with a special walker (U-step) designed for individuals with Parkinson's for whom balance and difficulty initiating and stopping movement is a primary symptom. This was prescribed by my neurologist after I had several falls weekly and one fall that required an ER visit. I can no longer drive. My attention and concentration skills are variable and range from not being able to concentrate on even a mindless activity such as watching a TV program or listening to music to about 1 hour of productive concentration to pay bills on line. My manual dexterity, due to increased tremors and dyskinesia, is poor and at best I can write a few words with poor legibility. Typing and navigating on the computer is laborious and frustrating. Text to speech programs have not been successful to compensate for these difficulties.

The pain I experience from PN has become considerably worse over the last 18 months despite physicians' continued best efforts to control it with medication and non-pharmacological interventions, e.g., meditation. I feel constant pain in my feet, which requires me to keep off of my feet as much as possible. The frequency and duration of episodes of intense pain which are debilitating has increased—all I can do is lie in bed until the pain subsides. While there is variation in days, I typically need to spend at least an hour in bed after finishing breakfast, 2 or more hours in the afternoon and again an hour or more after dinner.

I was diagnosed with lymphoma in April, 2013, but my lymphoma is indolent and has not yet had an impact on my daily life.

Question 2.
Please list all of the types of activities you do during the course of a typical day. What do you specifically do from the time you arise in the morning until you retire at night? Do you require assistance with any of your daily activities?

My ability to participate in daily activities has significantly declined. I can walk short distances using a specialized walker most of the time and a cane with the support of another person some of the time. I can no longer drive. I can read for at most 15 minutes and have transitioned to audiobooks. I continue to try to use e-mail but it takes me an inordinate amount of time to compose and produce even a short message. I continue to talk on the phone occasionally. I have further reduced the amount of time I spend doing volunteer work for the one charity I am currently associated with due to fatigue, my PN foot pain and my diminished ability to concentrate.

My wife assists me in getting out my clothes, occasional supervision while showering for safety, meal preparation, and ambulation. She performs most household tasks the majority of the time as I can only occasionally assist with dishes or taking out the garbage. I am responsible for paying bills but as mentioned earlier it takes me much longer than the average person.

Question 3.
Please provide the following information about the condition causing your disability. Next to any Activity of Daily Living (ADL) please place the number shown next to the statement that most accurately reflects your ability/inability to perform each of them.

Dress—1, but need assistance getting clothes out
Toilet—1
Bathe—2, shower seat and hand held shower head; occasional supervision for safety
Voluntary bladder and bowel control—2, incontinent, use pad day and night
Feed self—1, but increased difficulty due to tremors and dyskinesia

Transfer from bed to chair—1

I have experienced increased cognitive impairment over the last 18 months which is demonstrated by forgetfulness in taking medications on time even with use of audible reminder.

Question 4.

What kinds of hobbies or social/community activities did you engage in prior to your disability?

Activities I did before my disability included working, running, hiking, playing catch, bicycling, going to movies and concerts, and volunteer work for charitable organizations.

At this point I can no longer work, run, hike, do any physical game-like activity or bicycle outdoors. I participate in a Pedaling for Parkinson's group at the local YMCA 2-3x per week but am unable to comply with the protocol as it creates such fatigue I am unable to participate in any activities the rest of the day and even part of the next day. I no longer go to movies as I cannot sit for that long and rarely go to an event such as a concert for the same reason. Evening activities are usually not a possibility as I am too fatigued and in pain at that time. I have cut back my volunteer activity to one organization and play a limited role.

Please fax the completed form to:

ATTENDING PHYSICIAN'S STATEMENT - PROGRESS REPORT

To be completed by the Employee

Patient Name:	Date of Birth:	Insured ID Number:
IRA FRIED		

Patient Address: (Street, City, State & Zip Code)

Ann Arbor, MI 48103

To be completed by the Provider - Use current information from your patient's most recent office visit or examination to complete this form. (The patient is responsible for the completion of this form without expense to the Company.)

Medical Conditions Impacting Activity

Primary condition: PARKINSONS   ICD-9 Code: 3320
ICD-10 Code:

Secondary condition(s): _____ Parkinson Neuropathy   ICD-9 Code: 333.9
ICD-10 Code(s):

Subjective symptoms:

Objective Physical Findings (Please include office notes for date(s): ___ to ___
Reduced Balance, Dyskinesia

Pertinent Test Results (list all results or attach test results):

Test _____ Date: _____ Results: _____

Test _____ Date: _____ Results: _____

Condition(s) Specific Medications, Dosage and Frequency: _____

TREATMENT PLAN

Current Treatment Plan: _____

What is the Frequency / Duration of Treatment? _____ Dates of Treatment: _____
First Office Visit for this condition: 3/2014 Last Office Visit: 5/27/16 Next Scheduled Office Visit: 5/4/16
Has Surgery been performed since last report? ☐ Yes ☒ No If "Yes," on what Date(s): _____
Procedure(s): _____ CPT Code(s): _____
Was patient hospitalized since last report? ☐ Yes ☒ No If "Yes," Hospital name and Phone Number: _____
_____ Admission date: _____ Discharge date: _____
Has patient been referred to other physicians? ☐ Yes ☒ No If "Yes," Date of Referral(s): _____

Other Physician Name _____ Phone Number: ( ) _____ Specialty: _____
Other Physician Name _____ Phone Number: ( ) _____ Specialty: _____

LC-7137-10   Page 1 of 2   08/2015

Patient Name: _CRYT PRIES_   Date of birth: _____   Insured ID Name: _____

Please complete this section to the best of your ability. Generalized comments such as 'unable to work', may delay your patient's disability benefits.

Based on your most recent medical findings and opinion, address the full range of restrictions/limitations, noting that we will conclude there are no restrictions on function unless specified below.

Restrictions/Limitations based on office visit dated: _____   Expected Return to Work date: _____

In an 8 hour period the patient is able to: (select either continuous or intermittent)

	Continuously with standard breaks		Intermittently with standard breaks	If intermittent circle time for each section below		
				Hours at one time		Total hours/8 hours
Sit	☐	or	☐	1 2 3 4 5 6 7 8	1 2 3 4 5 6 7 8	
Stand	☐	or	☐	1 2 3 4 5 6 7 8	1 2 3 4 5 6 7 8	
Walk	☐	or	☐	1 2 3 4 5 6 7 8	1 2 3 4 5 6 7 8	

Provide medical finding/rationale for your opinion if patient is unable to continuously sit, stand or walk:

Activity Ability (with normal breaks)	Never 0 hours	Occasionally up to 2.5 hours	Frequently 2.5 to 5.5 hours	Constantly 5.5 to 8 hours	Please indicate diagnosis, symptoms, exam findings, and/or imaging that supports the restrictions/limitations
Bend at waist	☐	☐	☒	☐	
Kneel/crouch	☐	☐	☒	☐	
Climb	☒	☐	☐	☐	
Balance	☒	☐	☐	☐	
Drive	☒	☐	☐	☐	
Lift - Indicate weight in pounds		_20_ lbs.	___ lbs.	___ lbs.	
Other Restrictions (if any)	☐	☐	☐	Requires 2 naps /day

Hand Dominance: ☐ Right ☐ Left

Upper Extremity Activity (not load bearing) Specify right (R) or left (L) if not bilateral

Fine manipulation (fingering, keyboard)	☒	☐	☐	☐	
Gross manipulation (grip/grasp, handle)	☐	☐	☐	☐	
Reach (extend arms) above shoulder	☐	☐	☐	☐	
Reach (extend arms) below shoulder at desk or workbench level	☐	☐	☐	☐	

Please attach copies of imaging results/tests

Expected duration of any restriction(s) or limitation(s) listed above: _Life long_

Current Status (Please check one): ☐ Recovered ☐ Improved ☐ Unchanged ☒ Retrogressed

Additional Comments (if necessary): _the Seizure Neurotoxic plus – medications_
lessened to control loss cognard

Does the patient have a psychiatric / cognitive impairment? ☒ Yes ☐ No If "Yes," please describe the extent of the impairment and its etiology: _Some Memory problems_

In your opinion is the patient competent to endorse checks and direct the use of the proceeds? ☒ Yes ☐ No

Provider's Name: (please print or type) _____   EIN Number: _____   License Number: _____

Telephone Number: _____   Fax Number: _____   Degree: _M.D._   Specialty: _Neurology_

Street Address: _____   _Ann Arbor, MI 48109_

Office Contact and Telephone Number: _____

_6/22/12_
Date signed

LC-7537-10   Page 2 of 2   09/2015

CHAPTER 25
TO BE OR NOT TO BE

I was wrong to think of myself as a fraud, as I described myself earlier in this memoir. The affable, confident guy who seemed to take his diseases in stride was no less the real me than the husband and father who often stayed up late at night worrying about what was to become of his family and himself. We all play many different roles each day: proud parent on the sidelines cheering on his child, athlete in training, mid-level executive dressing up for an important meeting with senior management, and so on. We may act and dress differently for our different roles. But in each role we remain our whole, true selves.

As many as 50 percent of the people with Parkinson's, possibly more, suffer from clinical depression. (This number is based on a cursory review of websites devoted to Parkinson's and/or mental illness. Estimates vary greatly, from a low of 40 percent to as high as 90 percent. It is difficult to come up with a precise estimate because there are few peer-reviewed, scholarly articles on the topic. Also, many cases go unreported.) I am one of the lucky ones. Most of the time, during the day, I do not feel depressed. I am too focused on what I am doing in the here and now. As long as I stay busy I am able to out-run my depression.

But a few times a week, almost always in the afternoon after I have slowed down, my thoughts wander from the present to fears of the future and regrets about the past.

Feelings of guilt, remorse, uselessness, and fear wash over me. The depressed Ira thinks and acts differently from the confident, upbeat persona I project in public, so much so that I sometimes feel as if I am living a double life. But I realize that the public and private me are both my whole, true self.

Depression is not new to me. It has been an unwelcome companion for as long as I can remember. During my childhood, depression hung over me all the time. I wore it like an old, frayed, dirty shirt, always there for everyone to see. There was no discernible difference between my public and private selves. But somehow, near the end of my senior year in high school, I found the strength and self-discipline to take off the shirt and put it in a box, which I placed on a shelf somewhere deep in the recesses of my memory. The box, always within reach but hardly ever in view, remained a deep, dark secret to all but my closest friends.

I naively thought after my success in college that I had vanquished my childhood demons. I could throw out the shirt I had once so shamefully worn. And why not? I was, after all, "The man with a future," as a friend called me after I received an acceptance letter from Northwestern's economics PhD program. I had a wide circle of friends. Women seemed to take an interest to me. I had run a 3:05 marathon and a sub-five-minute mile. And most precious to me, I had achieved a 3.94 grade point average and earned all the honors that went along with it.

Popular among both men and women, widely recognized by both my peers and faculty as one of the top undergraduate students at Fordham, and a legitimate athlete, I had succeeded in every realm important to me. But the sense of well-being these accomplishments gave me proved to be surprisingly frail and ephemeral.

My childhood demons, very much alive, bubbled just below the surface. There they were: feelings of inadequacy, being alone in the world with no place to call home, and wondering if I could ever love and if anyone would ever love me. All it took was for my girlfriend in San Francisco to break up with me for these feelings to crash through to the surface, as if a dam that had held them back had suddenly collapsed. I was lost. To paraphrase Bob Dylan once again, I had no direction home.

But then a remarkable series of events lifted me out of my depression and changed my life. First, I discovered that my randomly assigned roommate at Northwestern shared my love for running as well as my intellectual curiosity. Jim and I discussed everything, from each other's PhD programs to the meaning of life. In short order, we became close friends.

Two weeks after I arrived at Northwestern, convinced that I was condemned to a life of solitude and despair, I attended a party for the first-year graduate students. I stood by myself thinking I should probably go back to my room soon when I felt a light touch on my shoulder. I turned around and saw before me a beautiful woman with shoulder-length brown hair, doey brown eyes and a smile that rained sunshine on my dark mood. She stood about 5'6" and had a slim athletic body. Joy introduced herself and said she recognized my voice from high school. She not only recognized me but seemed to have liked me. How could I have failed to notice her?

A relationship that started with a weekly racquet ball game blossomed into a friendship that became the foundation of the love, respect, and affection we have felt for each other for the last thirty-five years.

Last and most improbable, in my first days at Northwestern I received a note that had been tucked into a letter from my stepsister. From my third-grade best friend for life, Cliff, it stated simply he was glad to hear I was alive. I hadn't seen Cliff since the summer after fourth grade, when my family moved away from Lexington to Pittsfield, Massachusetts. Why had he chosen the words "You're alive!"? His note made me realize I did have something to live for at a time when I was questioning my reason for being.

Over the next ten-plus years I suffered several bouts of depression, each time feeling the same sense of worthlessness I felt as a child, and again when I started at Northwestern. Joy urged me to seek professional help but I ignored her, preferring the misery depression brought on to the stigma of being treated for a mental illness. But finally I relented. My therapist taught me how to use Cognitive Behavioral Therapy, which along with a daily 20 milligram dose of Celexa helped me overcome the negative thinking that had so often brought me down.

For the next fifteen years or so depression rarely entered my life. My sense of well-being during these years was buttressed by the knowledge that in Joy and my children I had someone to love and someone to love me. I had also found my direction home: any place where I am with Joy. For now and probably the rest of my life that place is Ann Arbor.

I lived a charmed life during my first few years in Ann Arbor. I loved my job and was regularly rewarded as a top performer. I worked out with "The Group" every Wednesday evening, and I fully participated in Alan's and Sam's lives as they grew up. It was a magical time for me.

My outlook on life remained positive even after the Parkinson's diagnosis. Without intending to, I used denial as my primary coping mechanism, rarely giving much thought to the long-term consequences of the disease.

Two years later I was diagnosed with peripheral neuropathy and a year after that with kidney cancer. That made me wonder: *Am I being punished for something? How could I have been so lucky at Northwestern and so unlucky thirty years later? Was a sometimes benevolent, sometimes malevolent being looking after me?*

I had struggled with questions such as these since, as a twelve-year-old, I had rejected my religious upbringing and religion in general. I had nothing to believe in to help me deal with this crisis.

Not until three days before I was scheduled to have my kidney removed did I have the lightning-bolt moment of insight that wove my disparate thoughts into a cohesive belief system. This helped me to make sense of it all. It gave me the strength to weather the early storms of my diseases.

The mass in my kidney proved to be one of the seven percent of its type to be benign. However, not two years later I was diagnosed with another cancer: non-Hodgkin's lymphoma.

My belief system, CBT, Celexa, a weekly visit to a psychologist, plus—and most important—a heavy dose of denial, helped me to keep my depression under control. But as my neuropathy pain grew worse it became too much to ignore. I could no longer deny it. Stripped of the layer of protection denial had afforded me, I became vulnerable to my long-hidden fears for the future and regrets of the past.

. . . .

Sometimes my neuropathy pain is almost unbearable. The pain is centered at the base of my pointer toes, left always worse than my right. During a moderately painful episode, both types of pain can spread all the way to the balls of my feet. During more extreme episodes the falling asleep sensation travels to my thighs and sometimes up to the trunk of my body. Occasionally, I can even feel the tingling in my head.

The medical professions use a ten-point scale for patients to self-report pain. One means no pain and ten means the worst pain imaginable. My worst neuropathy pain episodes hit eight and a half to nine on this scale. At this level the pain completely overwhelms me. I lie in bed unable to do anything. I have no desire to watch TV or listen to music. I don't want to talk to anyone. The only thing that helps is Joy lying on the bed next to me.

These episodes scare me almost as much as they hurt. Something akin to an electrical shock courses from my toes up to my head at least a couple of times during each of these episodes. Remembering that my father died of a massive heart attack at age fifty-one, I fear I am about to have one, too. So what if the tests on my own heart have all shown it to be healthy? The prospect of dying here and now scares me. But at the same time another voice in me welcomes death, even wishes it would come. Death would free me from pain, my responsibilities, and the horror that my condition will only get worse over time.

With some help from my therapist, I have learned to cope just a little better with these neuropathy pain episodes. I remind myself I have survived episodes like this before. And I tell myself over and over that the pain will not last forever. This too shall pass.

Fortunately, neuropathy pain episodes this bad are rare—perhaps once every few weeks. Far more common are episodes that reach seven on the ten-point pain scale. At that level I need to lie down in bed, but I can at least be semi-productive—I read, listen to my Audible books, occasionally watch TV—anything to avoid just lying there doing nothing. I can almost count on having one of these episodes each evening as I get ready for bed. Otherwise they're unpredictable. I don't know when they will come or how long they will last. They can last an hour. They can last for an entire day.

Neuropathy pain, more than any other symptom of my illnesses, has caused me to lose confidence in myself. I can never be sure when making a commitment whether neuropathy pain will force me to break it. Do I complain about it too much? Am I a coward for succumbing to it? I feel guilty even writing these words.

There are times when I have no recourse but to keep my commitment and fight through the pain. Not long ago Joy, the boys, and I had plans to go out to eat to celebrate Sam's eighteenth birthday. An episode started a couple of hours before our 6 p.m. reservation. I lay in bed, hoping the pain would subside before we got to the restaurant, but it only got worse. By the time we left the house it had reached eight on the ten-point scale. I hobbled the two blocks from our parking spot to the entrance just barely able to make it. The restaurant, an upscale New York-style bistro with an atmosphere of energy and exclusivity, had a line out the door. Perhaps noticing my ungainly entrance and seeing the desperation in my eyes, the hostess found a table for us right away. We snaked our way through a maze of tightly-knit tables and were seated at one just large enough to hold our dishes.

While Joy and the boys took in the crowded, busy atmosphere, I struggled to make myself comfortable. I took off my shoes and put them under my chair—the only space available—then with Joy's help, figured out a safe way to stow my cane.

Having settled in, Joy and the boys started up a conversation about the relative merits of books, movies, and TV shows they had recently read or watched. I sat at the table writhing in pain, trying to find a comfortable position in our cramped quarters. I tried my best to hide my pain but found it hard to think of anything else. On a few rare occasions I managed to say something that contributed to the conversation.

The pain started to subside, just a little, as we got up to leave the restaurant. It continued to ease and by the time we got home about fifteen minutes later it had gone down to about six and a half. I had found the strength to fight through it and participate in this important event in Sam's life. But I hadn't participated; I was just there. I felt not one iota of satisfaction for my "accomplishment."

Sometimes depression washes over me without any provocation. I feel it as a fog enveloping me and my thoughts. Often, I can see it coming, but I can't do anything to stop it or escape from it. I feel a deep despair that leads me to ask myself the existential questions: *What has been the meaning of my life? Have I accomplished anything worthwhile? Am I contributing anything worthwhile now? Or am I just taking up space, using resources that could be better spent on other people?*

Sure, I tried to help others by serving on non-profit boards, but my time for playing an active role in these organizations is over. When MAP's board president called to ask whether I would be interested in chairing a new board committee charged with updating MAP's three year-old strategic plan, I dove right into the assignment.

I got the committee off to a good start but soon found my energy waning. I simply could not keep up with the back and forth emails needed to keep the committee on track. Each time I planned to get re-engaged and provide some leadership, a neuropathy pain episode stopped me.

If I could no longer lead a committee for one of the four organizations to which I had once been indispensable, what could I do? The answer stared me right in the face, but I could not see it through the fog of depression that surrounded me.

First, I asked Joy. She reminded me there are many

other ways of helping people. "Why not try to find something you actually enjoy doing?" she suggested. She also told me she could not imagine living without having me in her life. Next, I asked Jim. He urged me to focus on completing my memoir. It will make a difference in the lives of those closest to me. And it could be my legacy to future generations of my family. Finally, I asked my therapist. She told me how damaging my committing suicide would be to the rest of my family; she disabused me of any notion I would get a bye because my children are nearly grown.

These conversations helped me to see through the haze. I could see clearly I have far too much to do to consider suicide. I need to be present for Alan and Sam as they struggle to find their way from adolescence to independent adulthood—they are, after all, my most important legacy. I need to continue to be Joy's companion, best friend, and confidante. And I need to finish writing my memoir so others might benefit from my experiences.

My *It's a Wonderful Life* epiphany helped me to rediscover what is most important to me. However, my depression persists. My doctors cannot remove it with a scalpel as they did the mass in my kidney. It permeates my very being. Each morning I face a brand new challenge, trying to get myself out of bed. It would be so much easier to just lie there under my warm, comfortable covers.

What gives me the wherewithal to get out of bed each and every morning? I think willpower plays an important role. Each morning I tell myself I must move; I must drag myself out of bed to start the new day. I try to remind myself of Woody Allen's quote: "Eighty percent of being a person is just showing up."

Also, I am lucky to have a short memory when it comes to pain. My neuropathy episodes always feel worse in the moment than they do in the rearview mirror. Perhaps that is why I always came back for more at school despite knowing I could expect another day of taunting and abuse.

But I think, more than anything else, I am too curious and hopeful about what the next day will bring to stay in bed. Who knows what will happen today in this beautiful, random world in which we live? I don't want to miss out if something good happens. I know I need to be present to take advantage of my good luck.

Not long ago my neurologist told me about the Pedaling for Parkinson's program at the Ann Arbor YMCA. The program is part of a follow-up to a study done a few years ago at the Cleveland Clinic that demonstrated pedaling a bicycle at high RPMs several times a week can slow and possibly stop progression of the disease. I had heard of the program before but decided not to join because I thought my peripheral neuropathy pain would prevent me from cycling and/or the cycling would make the pain worse. But this time, with my doctor's encouragement, I decided to give it a try.

The program has been an unexpected gift, its value immeasurable. Over the last ten years since my Parkinson's forced me to stop running marathons, I have gradually reduced the intensity of my workouts. I cannot fix a date on it but I have long since given up any pretensions of being an athlete. My workouts have become merely light aerobic exercise, something everyone should do a few times each week to stay healthy. I discovered just a few minutes after getting on the bike for the first time that the Peddling for Parkinson's workouts are hard—very hard. The study tracks each participant's heart rate, as well as the RPMs of his or her bike. Riders have to set the resistance at a high enough level to reach and maintain the desired heart rate. No coasting downhill here.

I got off the bike exhausted, drenched with sweat, and elated. I hadn't felt this way in years, since I used to rush out of my office every Wednesday to get to The Group's work-outs on time. Then in another of those seemingly unlikely coincidences that have shaped my life, I learned that Seanna, the woman who had been so welcoming the first day I ran with The Group, would be leading the next Pedaling for Parkinson's workout.

These workouts, with Seanna leading them, have given an important part of my life back to me. How incredibly lucky I am that this program exists at the Ann Arbor Y, less than a fifteen minute drive from our house. But I also made my own luck. I had to show up and give the program a try. Who knows how long I will be able to continue with it? Already, I have had to push through my neuropathy pain to get on the bike on several occasions.

I know now I am no longer the person I used to be. I have come full circle. I have learned once again that "All I can do is do what I must." So "I'll do what I must do and I'll do it well."

And so my journey continues ...

EPILOGUE
A RUN THROUGH PARADISE

Eight months after our wedding, Joy and I relocated from Chicago to Minneapolis, a move that presented a great opportunity to further my career. I had accepted a position as Consultant at Touche Ross (now Deloit and Touche), which meant I would be working for a prestige firm in a hot-bed of the nascent managed care industry. My starting salary, $45,000, was almost twice what Blue Cross Blue Shield Association paid me just three and a half years earlier, when I started my professional career.

Almost immediately, I began a project working on a start-up HMO for one of the two hospitals in Minot, North Dakota, working crazy hours. I usually traveled two days a week; on each of those days I worked about sixteen hours. Days in the office were shorter but more intense. I got into the office at 8:30 hoping that none of the managers noticed me arriving so late. Most days I went out to pick up something for lunch, which I brought back to my desk so I could continue working until I left the office at 7:30. When I got home, Joy and I told each other about our days while I changed into my running gear.

I ran no matter how bad the weather, including some evenings when the temperature dropped well below zero degrees. While I ran, Joy prepared dinner. After the run, I arrived back home at about nine. We usually ate and watched TV together until ten before going upstairs to get ready for bed.

Joy found a job shortly after the move. She worked forty hours a week, but also commuted an hour each way—and took responsibility for most of the household chores. My main responsibility was cleaning the dishes.

Life seemed hard. Joy and I often complained about how much time we spent working and how little time we had to ourselves and for each other. Occasionally at my office, when the workload seemed insurmountable, someone muttered the refrain popular at the time: "Life's a bitch and then you die." It was worth a chuckle the first time I heard it, but after that it just made me feel worse about my situation.

But Joy and I had no idea how good we had it. We chose the life we were living. Our only responsibilities were to ourselves and each other. We had just bought our first house, a beautiful brick colonial. We missed our friends and family from back East, but at least we were able to visit every year. Both of us athletes, we enjoyed excellent health and we treated ourselves to a nice vacation every year.

Our trips were the high point of the year for me. I relished planning them almost as much as I did going on them. Usually we spent our vacations sightseeing and hiking. I made sure we saw every site in the guidebook, which meant we raced from place to place, often coming home more tired than before we left.

But this time we agreed to find a resort where we could kick back and relax. We chose Antigua, a small Caribbean island with not much to offer besides warm, sunny weather and miles of gorgeous beaches. The only "site" of any interest to me was St. John's, the biggest city on the island, with a population of just over 25,000.

Joy and I had a history of bad luck with weather on our vacations and this trip was no exception. We got in late the first evening and didn't plan to do much, so the steady downpour did not dampen our spirits. Having awakened the first morning to a steady pitter-patter of rain on the roof, we decided to spend our first day sight-seeing. We ate a leisurely breakfast and then hired a taxi to take us to St. John's. After a short wait, the car arrived and we squeezed in. Joy and another couple sat in the back. I contorted my body into the front passenger seat, which I shared with a cooler filled with bottles of cold water. We bumped along the entrance to our resort for 300 yards or so until we reached the main road, a two-lane asphalt highway with a narrow gravel shoulder that ran parallel to the beach. As we sped along and cars zoomed by in the opposite direction, it became abundantly clear to me I would need to find a different road if I were to run on this island.

Upon our arrival in St. John's, I saw a tableau of empty stores that could have been the set for a *Dawn of the Dead* movie. Store after empty store, in the middle of the day, at the height of tourist season. I wondered how the island could survive with no one to buy all the stuff in the stores. Then the cruise ships arrived, first one, then another, then another still. Within an hour, all three ships had sidled up to the pier. They were enormous, easily dwarfing every building in St. John's.

Within minutes of arriving, the ships started to disgorge their passengers, first in a trickle, then in a steady stream, transforming St. John's from lonely outpost to frenetic marketplace. People ran, shouted, and bumped into each other, and most important, pulled out their wallets. The hungry mob, starved from not having had a chance to shop since leaving another island the previous day, first raced to the liquor and T-shirt stores closest to the ships. Then the more intrepid among them squeezed through the crowd and moved on to more expensive stores. A few wandered into shops selling local art. Most rushed into the fine jewelry stores. I saw more than a few men pull wads of cash from their wallets before engaging in what looked like heated discussion with the store owners. I presumed these men were negotiating the steals they would brag about to their table mates over dinner that night.

. . . .

Our resort arranged activities for its guests throughout the day. My favorite was volleyball. By the time we returned from St. John's, the rain had let up enough for me to check out the court—really no more than a net and some lines in the sand. Joy decided she had had enough rain and went up to our room to read.

I thought I might not get a chance to play, but a group of teenagers and some resort staff suddenly showed up. Now we had plenty of people. But a half hour later the rain picked up and most of the teenagers left. Now we needed one more player. Just as we were about to call it a day, a guy who had been cleaning the boats said he would join us. This man did not wear the standard issue shirt the rest of the resort staff wore. His had a beach scene surrounded by large black letters that read "Life's a Beach and Then You Dive."

After the game ended, I walked over to him and told him I liked his shirt.

He replied, "Thank you. It fits me just right." He walked away before I could formulate any questions about his shirt. But, intrigued by the man, I kept an eye out for him during the rest of our time at the resort. I also combed through area shops trying to find the shirt. But I found neither.

I went back to our room, where Joy sat on the bed reading. We bemoaned the bad weather and joked that countries suffering from drought should pay us to visit— any place we went on vacation was sure to have rain while we were there.

By the time we finished eating dinner, the rain had dissipated to a light drizzle. Joy and I went for a long walk on the beach and then got ready for bed. I did not have a chance to run, but I had gotten plenty of exercise, so I was happy.

. . . .

The next morning I woke up and pulled back the shades. I saw nothing but gray sky. But at least it was not raining. Joy and I checked the forecast on our daily activities sheet and were relieved to find out that the front causing all the bad weather was expected to pass by early that afternoon. Then it would be sunny for the next three days. Joy had wanted to get a facial and I wanted to go for a long run, so the overcast skies presented a perfect opportunity for both of us. I just needed to find a dirt road without too much traffic, where it would be safe to run.

I jogged down the entrance drive from our resort to the main road and turned right, away from St. John's. Then I got lucky. After only a quarter mile of death-defying running on the main road, a dirt road appeared on my left. I was in a runner's paradise—a warm overcast day on a dirt road with no traffic. The road seemed to stretch on forever, up and down gentle hills. After two miles or so, I came upon a tiny ramshackle village with ten to twelve shacks. The shabby homes, made of stucco and sheet metal, looked like they could easily be blown apart the next time a hurricane passed through. The village was strewn with garbage. Next to each shack was a small vegetable garden no more than twenty by forty feet wide. One house was completely open in the front.

At that house, two elderly men sat on crates, drinking. One of them raised his can in a greeting to me. I grunted something between Hi and Hello and picked up my pace. I wondered how people could live like that. A couple of women were tending their gardens. I started a "hello" but neither of them looked up to greet me.

A couple of miles ahead, I came upon a much larger village. As I entered it, I heard children chanting. I could clearly tell their words were directed at me but I could not make out what they were saying. I got closer and the chanting grew louder, but I still couldn't understand them. *The children must be happy to see me—they are welcoming me to their home,* I thought, *cheering me on.* As I approached, I smiled and readied my arm to wave until I heard what they were saying: "Run to your death, run to your death." Stunned by their words, I quickly turned around and raced back toward my hotel.

· · · · · · · · ·

A shock of fear coursed through my entire being. Not until I passed through the first, tiny village, head down, avoiding any eye contact, was I able to think a cogent thought. *Why were those children chanting "run to your death?" Why do they hate me? They don't even know me. I never did anything to hurt them.*

It took a while longer for me to think about the T-shirt again. Every once in a while, often while running, a thought about the shirt would pop up. What was the point? Was it just some words, or did it mean something? Then it came to me. Here are people living at subsistence wages, working terrible hours, and living on small farms to get by, and I'm running through their island as if I owned it. I also thought I was better than all the other people on the cruise who, after their frantic shopping, bragged to each other about the steals they had gotten on the island.

Then I started thinking about the man wearing the shirt. Why was he wearing it? Was he trying to send a message to the wealthy tourists who visited the island? Those who had cashed in on the islanders' despair? Or maybe it was just something he used to have a positive attitude, despite his circumstances. Or maybe he just needed a T-shirt and this one happened to be in the bin at the store.

This man likely had much more to complain about than me. And he had good reason to resent me. And yet, he wore a T-shirt that uplifted my spirits by telling me life was good, even though we both knew there was plenty in this world that was far from alright. That is why I like to call myself and others Parkies, even though I know that Parkinson's is a serious disease. And that is also why I like to say it gets better every day, even though I know it won't.

I can't attribute specific meaning to the words "Life's a Beach and Then You Dive." It's not a philosophy to live by, or even a motto. It's nothing more than clever wordplay.

But over the years, I thought about the shirt and the chanting from time to time, and whether it had any meaning for my life. Not until I started writing this memoir did the meaning become clear. Yes, life can be difficult, but we can also do our best to enjoy it. That's the "Life's a Beach." But we can't just stay where we are. "And Then You Dive." I didn't realize it at the time, but life truly had been a beach for me, before my Parkinson's diagnosis. I am thankful I dove numerous times. And I'm glad Joy dove with me.

Life is really not such a bitch. In fact, most of the time, our lives are pretty good. Compared to the lives of the less fortunate, ours are like a day at the beach.

Ira Fried
August 2017

Acknowledgments

I would like to express my gratitude to the people who helped to make this book possible. First and foremost, thank you to my friend and editor, Nancy Nelson. Nancy offered to help when after four years and over 125,000 words into the project, my manuscript was too long, had several key omissions, and was highly disorganized in some places. Using only my words, Nancy helped me to fix what was wrong with my manuscript, all the while resisting my urge to review each chapter over and over again. If not for her intervention, I would still be telling friends my memoir would be done in about three to four months.

I owe a huge debt of gratitude to Jas Obrecht, my writing mentor and guru. I had not done any creative writing since high school and was dubious about my ability to write a memoir. I entered Jas' memoir class in May 2012. Jas told me I had the potential to become an outstanding writer. Over the succeeding five years, Jas' advice and encouragement has helped me to come closer to reaching this goal than I ever thought possible. He not only taught me how to write, equally important, he gave me confidence by telling me that I write with a voice that people will want to hear.

A heartfelt thank you to my sisters Edythe and Mandy for reading the first draft of the chapters on my parents and childhood and confirming that it was as bad as I remembered. A second thank you to Edythe for designing the cover art and book design.

Thanks to Jim Walsh for all the long talks we have taken searching for the meaning of life. Jim has been my most enthusiastic supporter since the project began and has given me great advice. Many of the thoughts in the "This I Believe" chapter and other sections where I contemplate religious themes came about as a result of discussions with Jim.

Thank you to Stephanie Paul of the American Parkinson's Disease Association for her support and encouragement. She believed in my memoir when I did not.

Thanks to my Aunt Dorothy for helping to fill in the blanks of what I knew of my father.

And finally, thank you to George Allen, John Azzolini, Mike Banks, Rosalie Denenfeld, Diane Laboda, Pat Davis, Nancy Shaw, and Jody Burton-Slowins, who have read all or part of the manuscript and given me helpful feedback.

CPSIA information can be obtained
at www.ICGtesting.com
Printed in the USA
BVOW09*1925170817
491897BV00001B/1/P